# Osteology

## for Dental Students

### THIRD EDITION

# Osteology
## for Dental Students

THIRD EDITION

**Nafis Ahmad Faruqi**

MBBS, MS, MNYAS (USA), Man of YK2 (USA)

Professor
Department of Anatomy
JN Medical College, AMU
Aligarh-202002, India

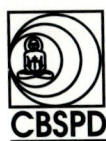

CBSPD

## CBS Publishers & Distributors Pvt Ltd

New Delhi • Bengaluru • Chennai • Kochi • Kolkata • Lucknow • Mumbai
Hyderabad • Jharkhand • Nagpur • Patna • Pune • Uttarakhand

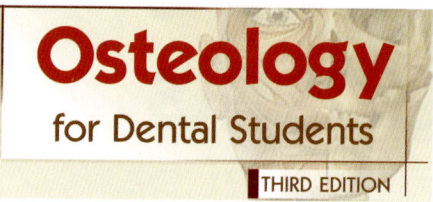

**ISBN:** 978-93-87085-19-0

**Third Edition: 2018**

Reprint: 2020, 2023

First Edition: 2001

Second Edition: 2011

Published by Satish Kumar Jain and Produced by Varun Jain for

**CBS Publishers & Distributors** Pvt Ltd

4819/XI Prahlad Street, 24 Ansari Road, Daryaganj, New Delhi 110 002, India
Ph: 011-23289259, 23266861

Website: www.cbspd.com
e-mail: delhi@cbspd.com

*Corporate Office:* 204 FIE, Industrial Area, Patparganj, Delhi 110 092, India
Ph: 011-4934 4934      Fax: 011-4934 4935      e-mail: publishing@cbspd.com; publicity@cbspd.com

*Branches*

• **Bengaluru:** Seema House 2975, 17th Cross, K.R. Road, Banasankari 2nd Stage, Bengaluru 560 070, Karnataka, India
Ph: +91-80-26771678/79      Fax: +91-80-26771680      e-mail: bangalore@cbspd.com
• **Chennai:** 7, Subbaraya Street, Shenoy Nagar, Chennai 600 030, Tamil Nadu, India
Ph: +91-44-26680620, 26681266      Fax: +91-44-42032115      e-mail: chennai@cbspd.com
• **Kochi:** 42/1325, 1326, Power House Road, Opp KSEB, Power House, Ernakulam 682 018, Kerala, India
Ph: +91-484-4059061-65,67      Fax: +91-484-4059065      e-mail: kochi@cbspd.com
• **Kolkata:** 147, Hind Ceramics Compound, 1st Floor, Nilgunj Road, Belghoria, Kolkata 700 056, West Bengal, India
Ph: +91-33-25633055/56      e-mail: kolkata@cbspd.com
• **Lucknow:** Basement, Khushnuma Complex, 7-Meerabai Marg (Behind Jawahar Bhawan), Lucknow 226 001, UP, India
Ph: 0522-4000032      e-mail: tiwari.lucknow@cbspd.com
• **Mumbai:** PWD Shed. Gala no. 25/26, Ramchandra Bhatt Marg, Next to JJ Hospital Gate no. 2,
Opp. Union Bank of India, Noorbaug Mumbai 400 009, Maharashtra, India
Ph: 022-66661880/89      e-mail: mumbai@cbspd.com

*Representatives*

| | | | | | |
|---|---|---|---|---|---|
| • **Hyderabad** | 0-9885175004 | • **Jharkhand** | 0-9811541605 | • **Nagpur** | 0-9421945513 |
| • **Patna** | 0-9334159340 | • **Pune** | 0-9923910676 | • **Uttarakhand** | 0-9716462459 |

*Printed at:* HT Media Ltd. Greater Noida, UP, India

*to*

---

*My father Late Jamil Ahmad Faruqi, my father-in-law Late Asloob Ahmad Ansari who left for heavenly abode before admiring my work. I would also like to dedicate to my beloved mother Sajida Khatoon, who will not be able to appreciate this book due to her illness. Talat Ara, my mother-in-law is the only person cherishing this special moment*

# Preface to the Third Edition

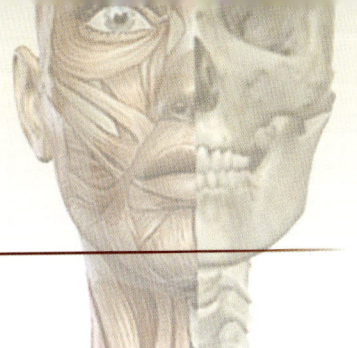

Third edition of **Osteology for Dental Students** has been thoroughly revised in the light of latest recommendations by Dental Council of India. The irrelevant material has been removed making the book more specific for dental students. All the diagrams have been redrawn and many new added by the author himself to ensure the accuracy. Coloured diagrams in this book have made it more fascinating. In the light of recent advances, additional applied anatomy has been incorporated in all the chapters. All these features will surely make the book palatable and more graspable.

A feedback from the readers will be highly appreciated to further improve the manuscripts in subsequent editions.

**Nafis Ahmad Faruqi**

Preface to the Third Edition

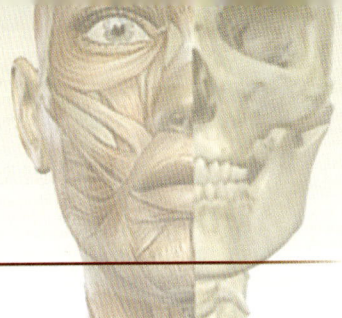

# Preface to the First Edition

**O**steology for Dental Students is a sort of gift to the dental undergraduate and postgraduate students. Descriptive details have been carefully monitored to make the book relevant for dental students. A unique feature of the book is the highly simplified illustrations which have been drawn by the author himself, minimizing the chances of the factual mistakes often discovered in the diagrams made by professional artists. Extremely precise treatment of the subject and clarity of linguistic expression are the focus of attention in this book.

The readers of the book are requested to kindly communicate to the author any shortcomings noticed by them and suggestions towards improvement when the book goes into subsequent editions.

**Nafis Ahmad Faruqi**

## Reader's Comments

Dear Reader,

I will feel honoured if you spare a few minutes from your precious time and comment on this book. Your suggestions will go long way in improving this book in subsequent editions.

*Address*

**Dr. Nafis Ahmad Faruqi**
Gulfishan
Allahwali Kothi
Dodhpur, Civil Lines
Aligarh-202001
Mob. 9358256504
WhatsApp no. 7060888167
Email: drnafisahmad@rediffmail.com

# Acknowledgements

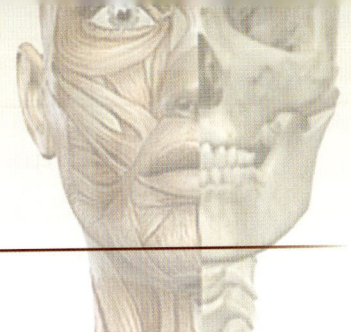

Publication of a book needs involvement of large number of persons, directly or indirectly. Coincidently 3rd edition of this book entitled *Osteology for Dental Students* came into existence, when our beloved colleague Professor Tariq Mansoor of department of surgery, became the Vice Chancellor of Aligarh Muslim University. I trust in his ability to run this great institution and wish him all the best.

Dr Krishna Garg, ex-Professor and Head, Department of Anatomy, Lady Hardinge Medical College, New Delhi, and chief editor of *BD Chaurasia's Human Anatomy*, vols 1–4 and author of many other books on anatomy, is the one who inspired me maximally during the period of my writing recent books. Her enthusiasm and vision have no match, not only in this country but all over the world. I really feel proud of being associated with her.

I do not have words to thank Prof Khursheed Alam, Professor and Head, Department of Anatomy, Patna Medical College, Patna, who liked my books and always encouraged me. His valuable advice was of great help in improving all my books in general and this book in particular. I feel obliged for promotion of my books by him among undergraduate as well as postgraduate students.

My special thanks to Dr SN Kazi (ex-Professor of Anatomy), Director, Kazi Medical Classes Academy and author of multiple books of anatomy, for his valuable suggestions which helped me in improving this book.

I am thankful to following individuals who not only personally took interest in my books but also recommended them to undergraduate and postgraduate students.

1. I am zero without the help of following members of CBS team, **Mr SK Jain** (*CMD*), **Mr YN Arjuna** (*Senior Vice President—Publishing, Editorial and Publicity*), **Mrs Ritu Chawla** (*AGM–Publishing)*, **Ms Ritu Tiwai** (*DTP Operator*), **Mr Sanjay Kishan Chauhan** (*Graphic Designer*), **Mr Neeraj Prasad** (*Cover and Graphic Designer*) and **Mr Kshirod Kumar Sahoo** (*Reader*)

2. Prof. Tabassum Shahab, Department of Paediatrics, JNMC, AMU, Aligarh, UP.

3. Prof. Mujahid Beg, Department of Medicine, JNMC, AMU, Aligarh, UP.

4. Prof. Shaista Vasenvala, Retired from Department of Pathalogy, JNMC, AMU Aligarh, UP.

5. Colleagues Prof. Tariq Zaidi (Head of the Department), Prof. Aijaz Ahmed Khan, Prof. SM Yunus, Dr SM Dawar Husain, Dr Farhan Kirmani, Dr Fazal Ur Rehman, Dr Farah Ghaus, Dr Nema Usman, Dr Mohd Imran, Dr Mohd Ajmal (SR), Dr Israr Ahmad Khan (SR), Dr Ragya Bharadwaj (SR).

6. **Postgraduate students:** Dr Pallavi Ranjan Anand, Dr Fayezah Ahsan Khan, Dr Mahammad Asif Khan, Dr Waqar Akram.

7. Dr Rati Tandon, Department of Anatomy, AIIMS, New Delhi
8. Dr Mohd Arshad, Department of Anatomy, Glocal Medical College, Superspeciality Hospital and Research Centre, Saharanpur, UP.
9. Prof. (Colonel) Arvind Kishor Shukla, Sena Medal, 529/228, Rashim Nagar, Mahanagar, Lucknow.
10. Prof. Navneet Sharma (Principal and Dean), Head, Department of Biochemistry, DJ College of Dental Science and Research, Modi Nagar, Ghaziabad, UP.
11. Dr (Mrs) Renu Agrawal, Department of Anatomy, DJ College of Dental Sciences and Research, Niwari Road, Modinagar, Ghaziabad, UP.
12. Dr Archana Tiwari, Head, Department of Anatomy, DJ College of Dental Sciences and Resarch, Niwari Road, Modi Nagar, Ghaziabad, UP.
13. Dr Mah Paiker, Tutor, Integral Institute of Medical Sciences and Research, Luknow, UP.
14. Dr Deeba Hasan, Senior Dental Surgeon, Motilal Nehra Divisional Hospital, Allahabad, UP.
15. Dr Shruti R Varshney, Senior Lacturer, KD Dental College, Mathura, UP.
16. Dr Sarah Mariam, Dental Surgeon, Flat No 2, Konark Indrayu Phase-2, NIBM Road, Kondhwa, Pune.
17. Dr Shakil Siddiqi (ex-Professor of Anatomy, KGMC and Era's Lucknow Medical College, Lucknow), 3/193, Vikas Khand, Gomti Nagar, Lucknow, UP.
18. Dr SH Hashmi, ex-Professor, Department of Oral and Maxillofacial Surgery, ex-Principal, Dr ZA Dental College, AMU, Aligarh, UP.
19. Dr Anand Mishra, Professor, Deptartment of Anatomy, IMS, BHU, Varanasi, UP.
20. Dr Naresh Chandra, Professor and Head, Department of Anatomy, Hind Institute of Medical Sciences, Safedabad, Barabanki, UP.
21. Dr Zeba Khan, Department of Anatomy, Grant Government Medical College and Sir JJ Group of Hospitals, Byculla, Mumbai, Maharashtra.
22. Prof. (Mrs) Geeta Rajput, Department of Prosthodontic/Dental Materials, Dr Ziauddin Ahmad Dental College, AMU, Aligarh, UP.
23. Prof. Syed Saeed Ahmad, Department of Oral and Maxillofacial Surgery, Dr Ziauddin Ahmad Dental College, AMU, Aligarh, UP.
24. Dr Shadab M Rizvi, Department of Oral and Maxillofacial Surgery, Dr Ziauddin Ahmad Dental College, AMU, Aligarh, UP.
25. Dr Ghulam Sarwar Hashmi, Department of Oral and Maxillofacial Surgery, Dr Ziauddin Ahmad Dental College, AMU, Aligarh, UP.
26. Dr Sajjad Abdur Rahman, Department of Oral and Maxillofacial Surgery, Dr Ziauddin Ahmad Dental College, AMU, Aligarh, UP.
27. Dr Kausar Jahan Khwaja, Department of Oral Pathology/Oral Medicine and Radiology, Dr Ziauddin Ahmad Dental College, AMU, Aligarh, UP.
28. Prof. ND Gupta, Department of Periodontia and Public Health Dentistry, Dr Ziauddin Ahmad Dental College, AMU, Aligarh, UP.
29. Prof. (Mrs) Afshan Bey, Department of Periodontia and Public Health Dentistry, Dr Ziauddin Ahmad Dental College, AMU, Aligarh, UP.
30. Dr Afaf Zia, Department of Periodontia and Public Health Dentistry, Dr Ziauddin Ahmad Dental College, AMU, Aligarh, UP.

31. Dr Saima Yunus Khan, Department of Paediatric and Preventive Dentistry, Dr Ziauddin Ahmad Dental College, AMU, Aligarh, UP.

32. Prof. (Mrs) Sandhiya Maheshwari, Department of Orthodontics and Dentofacial Orthopaedics, Dr Ziauddin Ahmad Dental College, AMU, Aligarh, UP.

33. Dr Sanjeev Kumar Verma, Department of Orthodontics and Dentofacial Orthopaedics, Dr Ziauddin Ahmad Dental College, AMU, Aligarh, UP.

34. Dr Mohammad Tariq, Department of Orthodontics and Dentofacial Orthopaedics, Dr Ziauddin Ahmad Dental College, AMU, Aligarh, UP.

35. Dr Syed Naved Zahid, Department of Orthodontics and Dentofacial Orthopaedics, Dr Ziauddin Ahmad Dental College, AMU, Aligarh, UP.

36. Dr Arbab Anjum, Department of Orthodontics and Dentofacial Orthopaedics, Dr Ziauddin Ahmad Dental College, AMU, Aligarh, UP.

37. Prof SK Mishra, Department of Conservative Dentistey and Endodontics, Dr Ziauddin Ahmad Dental College, AMU, Aligarh, UP.

37. Dr Sharique Alam, Department of Conservative Dentistey and Endodontics, Dr Ziauddin Ahmad Dental College, AMU, Aligarh, UP.

38. Dr Saba Khan, Department of Orthodontics and Dentofacial orthopaedics, Dr. Ziauddin Ahmad Dental College, AMU, Aligarh, UP.

39. Dr Upendra Kumar Gupta, Professor and Head, Department of Anatomy, National Institue of Medical Sciences and Research, NIMS University, Jaipur, Rajasthan.

40. Dr Rekha Parashar, Department of Anatomy, National Institue of Medical Sciences and Research, NIMS University, Jaipur, Rajasthan.

To my wife Roshan Ara, my children Arsalan Moinuddin and Anam Faruqi, daughter-in-law Siddiqua Abdullah and granddaughter Miss Fariha, I express my grateful appreciation for their patience, love, understanding and support.

**Nafis Ahmad Faruqi**

# Contents

# General Considerations of Bone

## DEFINITION

Bone is the hard part of the body providing dynamic framework to it.

## PROPERTIES

1. Bone is a living tissue.
2. Bone is supplied by arteries and nerves.
3. Bone is drained by veins.
4. Bone grows with age.
5. Bone is subject to disease.
6. Bone regenerates when damaged. It has greater regenerative power than any other tissue of the body, except blood.
7. Fractured bone heals leading to union.
8. Bone can undergo remodelling.
9. Bone can withstand strains and stresses.
10. Bone can atrophy or hypertrophy.

## FUNCTIONS

1. Bones provide framework to the body.
2. Bones accord shape to the body.
3. Bones act as levers for muscles and, therefore, help in the movements of the body.
4. Bones provide protection to number of viscera, e.g. brain, lungs and heart.
5. Bone is site of blood formation.
6. Bone plays important role in the immune responses of body by producing cells of reticuloendothelial system.
7. Bones are store houses of calcium and phosphorus.

## CHEMICAL COMPOSITION

Bone is one-third organic and two-thirds inorganic. Inorganic calcium salts [calcium phosphate, calcium carbonate and crystals of hydroxyapatite, i.e. $Ca_{10}\{PO_4\}_4(OH)_2$] make it hard and rigid. The organic connective tissue (collagen fibres) makes it tough and resilient. The collagen protein of collagen fibres is characterised by hydroxyproline amino acid.

## STRUCTURE OF BONE

### I. Macroscopically

There are two types of bones, *spongy* or *cancellous bone* and *compact* or *dense bone*. Outer part of all bones is made up of *compact bone* (Fig. 1.1). *Cancellous bone* fills up the interior of the bone except the following.

  i. In the shaft of long bone, it is replaced by *medullary cavity*. This is filled with *red marrow* in new born but replaced by *yellow* or *fatty marrow* in adults.

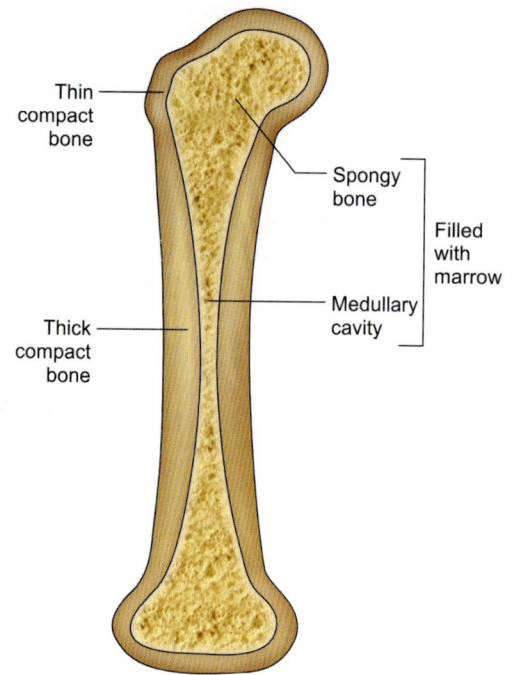

Fig. 1.1: Longitudinal section through a long bone

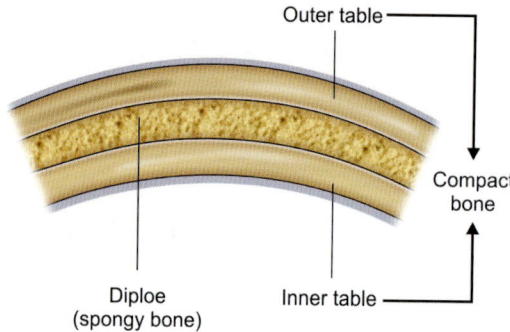

**Fig. 1.2:** Structure of the flat bone of calva

ii. In maxilla, sphenoid, ethmoid and frontal bones, it is replaced by large air spaces called *sinuses*.

iii. At many places the cancellous bone is replaced by marrow. The red marrow is active in hematopoiesis. Yellow marrow is mainly inert and fatty.

The flat bones of skull cap (calva) have spongy bone (*diploe*) sandwiched between two compact bones called *outer and inner tables* (Fig. 1.2). Red marrow persists in spongy bone throughout life.

The compact bone is more radio-opaque, while spongy bone is relatively more radiolucent. In radiograph, therefore, the compact bone looks more white than spongy bone which appears relatively darker.

## II. Microscopically

Microscopically the bones can be classified into four types:

i. *Lamellar bone:* Most of the mature human bones, both compact and spongy, are of this type.

ii. *Fibrous bone:* It is found in early foetuses.

iii. *Dentine:* It is found in teeth.

iv. *Enamel:* It is found in teeth.

The compact bone shows typical *Haversian systems* each of which is comprised of a central canal along the long axis of bone surrounded by *concentric lamellae. Volkmann's canals* connect the adjacent Haversian canals. *Osteocytes* are located in the small spaces (*lacunae*) between adjacent lamellae (Fig. 1.3). The cytoplasmic processes of osteocytes extend into *canaliculi* diverging from lacunae. *Circumferential lamellae* adjoin the surface or medullary cavity of long bones. *Interstitial lamellae* fill the spaces between Haversian systems.

Spongy bone differs from compact bone in 'lacking Haversian systems' and 'having irregularly arranged bony lamellae'

*Periosteum*, the outer covering of bone, consists of an external collagen fibrous layer and inner osteogenic cellular layer. Collagen fibres from periosteum piercing the bone are called *Sharpey's fibres*. Periosteum has a rich nerve supply which makes it most sensitive part of bone.

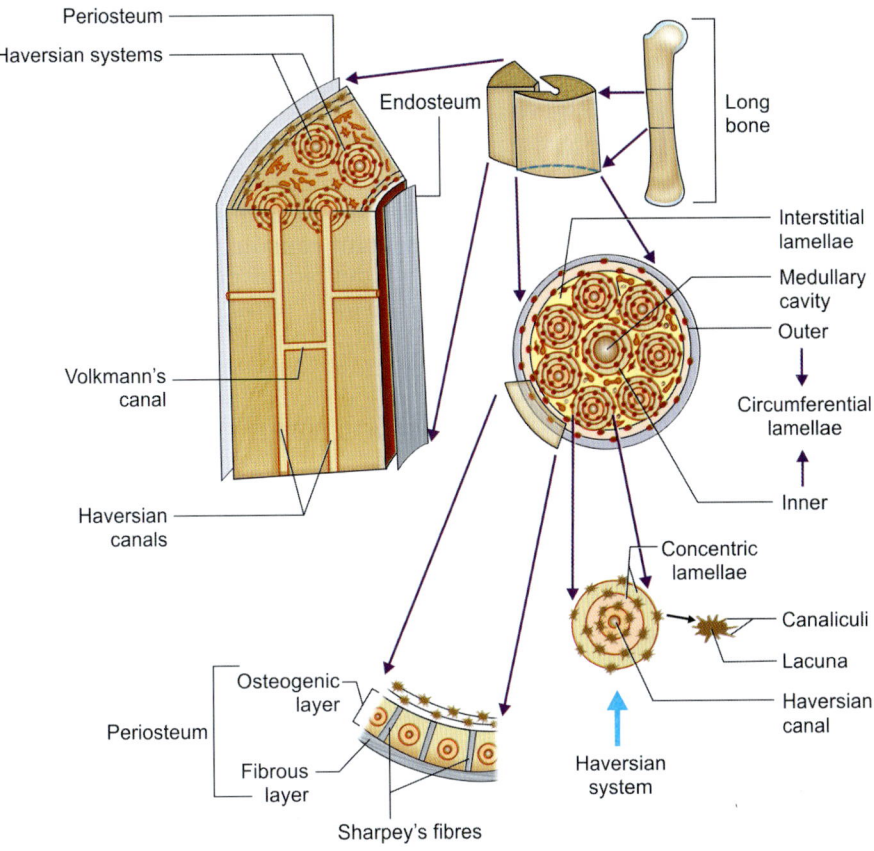

**Fig. 1.3:** Microscopic structure of compact bone

## CLASSIFICATION OF BONES

Bones may be classified according to their development, shape or location.

### I. Phylogenetic classification

From comparative anatomy point of view skeleton may be classified as:

#### a. Exoskeleton

Nails, hairs and enamel of teeth are the only remnants of exoskeleton observed in human being.

#### b. Endoskeleton

It includes most of the bones.

### II. Developmental classification

Developmentally bones may be classified as:
  a. *Cartilaginous bones*
  b. *Membranous bones*

### III. Morphological classification

According to shape, the bones may be classified as:

*a. Long bones* – Femur, humerus
*b. Short bones* – Carpal and tarsal bones
*c. Miniature long bones* – Metacarpals and metatarsals
*d. Flat bones* – Parietal bone
*e. Irregular bones* – Hip bone
*f. Pneumatic bones* – Maxilla, ethmoid, sphenoid and frontal bone.

## IV. Regional classification

Bones may be classified regionally as:

### a. Axial bones

It includes 80 bones as shown below.

| | | |
|---|---|---|
| i. Skull bones | – | 22 |
| ii. Vertebrae | – | 26 |
| iii. Ribs | – | 24 |
| iv. Sternum | – | 1 |
| v. Auditory ossicles | – | 6 |
| vi. Hyoid | – | 1 |

### b. Appendicular bones

It includes 126 bones which are further subgrouped as:

i. Upper limb bones – 64
ii. Lower limb bones – 62
   Total number of bones is 206

## V. Miscellaneous classification

### a. Accessory bones

An accessory bone is a small piece of bone which develops from a separate centre of ossification but fails to unite with the main mass of bone, e.g. sutural (Wormian) bones and interparietal bones (Fig. 1.4).

### b. Sesamoid bones

A sesamoid bone is a bone usually small, developing in the tendon of a muscle, ligament or joint capsule. They ossify after birth and are devoid of periosteum. Sesamoid bones possibly resist pressure, they alter the direction of pull of muscle and minimize the friction.

## BLOOD SUPPLY OF BONES

  I. **Short bones:** These are supplied by numerous periosteal vessels.
 II. **Vertebrae:** The body of vertebra is supplied by the anterior and posterior vessels (Fig. 1.5). The vertebral arch is supplied by large vessels entering through the bases of transverse processes.
III. **Ribs:** These are supplied by nutrient and periosteal vessels.

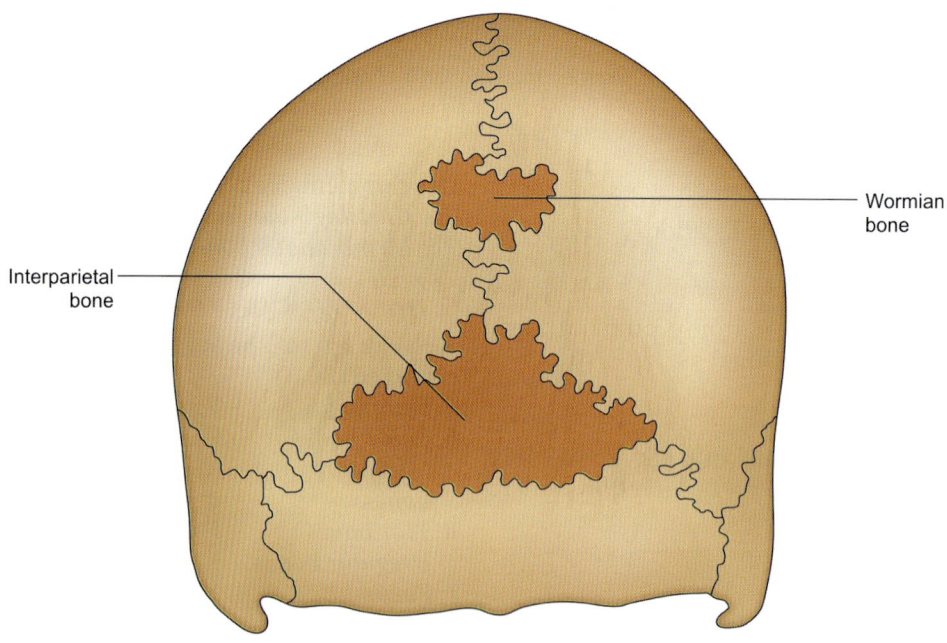

**Fig. 1.4:** Accessory bones

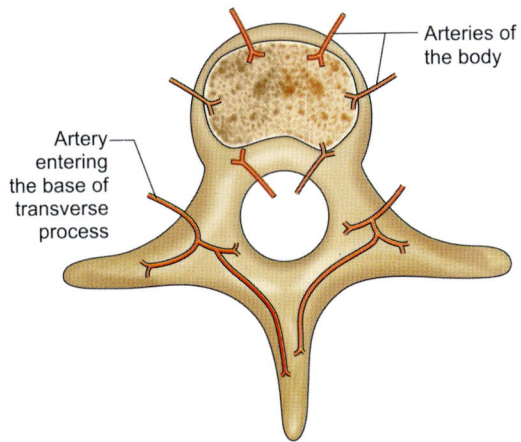

Arteries of the body

Artery entering the base of transverse process

**Fig. 1.5:** Arterial supply of vertebra

Here, the epiphysis usually appears earlier and fuses with the body later than that at the non-growing end.

## APPLIED ANATOMY OF BONES

1. Organic matter in the bone is greatest in childhood making it more flexible.
2. In *rickets* and *osteomalacia* there is inadequate calcium in bone leading to knock knees and bowlegs (Fig. 1.12).
3. Metaphysis is the commonest site of infection due to rich vascular anastomosis which has relatively less lymphocytes and has hairpin loop arrangement of blood vessels.
4. Capsular relations of metaphysis are clinically important. The inflammation of intra-articular metaphysis may result into septic arthritis, e.g. upper end of femur.
5. Injury of the growing ends of long bones is more dangerous in young children because it will directly affect the growth.
6. In certain conditions (e.g. *pernicious anaemia*) the yellow marrow is replaced by red marrow to enhance the formation of red blood cells.
7. Some interesting facts regarding fractures in young children are as follows:
   i. It is more common due to care-free activities.
   ii. *Green-stick fracture* (incomplete fracture with bending) is common in children due to excessive elasticity in bone.
8. In old age there is generalized skeletal atrophy called *osteoporosis* which makes the bone very weak. *Osteoporosis* is relatively more common in females, therefore, fracture of femoral neck is more common in elderly lady.
9. In *sternal puncture* the needle pierces the compact bone to reach central spongy bone from where red marrow is aspirated for haematological examination. The same procedure is used for bone marrow transplantation.

**IV. Flat bones:** These are supplied by nutrient and periosteal vessels.

## NERVE SUPPLY OF BONES

Nerves accompany the blood vessels of bone. Periosteal nerves are sensory (carry pain) while others are vasomotor in nature.

## LYMPHATIC DRAINAGE OF BONES

Lymphatics have not been demonstrated within bone but these are very much present in periosteum which drain into regional lymph nodes.

## OSSIFICATION OF BONES

1. Bones ossify from centres of ossification from where laying down of long lamellae starts by osteoblasts.
2. Centres of ossification may be primary or secondary. *Primary centre* appears before birth, usually during 8th week of intrauterine life and gives rise to diaphysis. *Secondary centre* appears at or after birth and gives rise to epiphysis.
3. Most of the long bones have *epiphysis* at each end but the growth in length occurs mainly at one end. This end is called *growing end*.

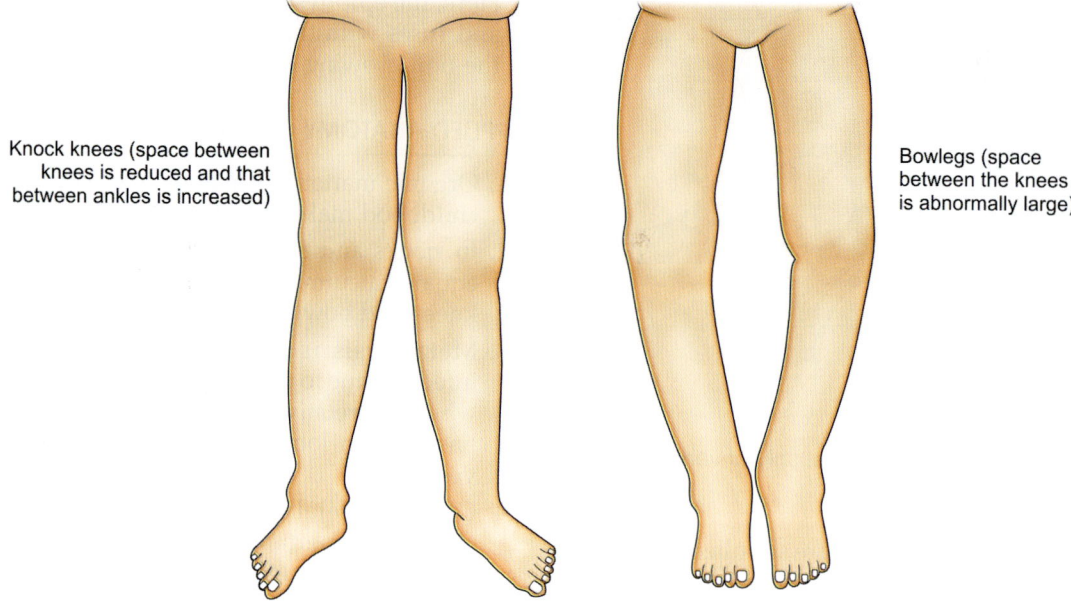

Knock knees (space between knees is reduced and that between ankles is increased)

Bowlegs (space between the knees is abnormally large)

**Fig. 1.6:** Deformities of the lower *limb* in *rickets* and osteomalacia

10. For perfect healing, the fractured ends of a bone should be properly aligned. This is called *reduction*. Healing is difficult and defective if the bony ends are mobile. To make them immobile, a hard cast is made around the fractured site and adjacent joints. This is called *plaster immobilization*.

11. Age of a person can be determined by observing the ossification centres of the bones and their fusion in the radiographs. This is of *medicolegal importance*.

12. Part of a bone may be deprived of blood supply after fracture. This leads to *avascular necrosis*. The best example of avascular necrosis is head of femur after fracture of neck.

13. Fibrous capsule is the most sensitive structure in a joint.

14. *Bone cyst* is the most common cause of pathological fracture in child.

15. Increased density in metaphysis is seen in *hypervitaminosis*.

16. *Senile osteoporosis* is radiologically manifested only when 30% of skeleton has been lost.

17. Multiple bone fracture in a newborn is seen in *osteogenesis imperfecta*.

18. Two interesting facts regarding *Ewing's tumour* are:

    a. It arises from diaphysis.

    b. It is very sensitive to radiotherapy.

# Skull: General Features

## INTRODUCTION (Fig. 2.1)

1. Skull is the skeleton of the head.

2. *Cranium* means skull minus the mandible.

3. *Neurocranium* is upper part of skull which encloses the brain

4. *Calvaria* is the upper part of the cranium. It is also called the skull cap.

5. *Facial skeleton (viscerocranium)* is skull minus the calvaria.

6. Facial skeleton is further divided into upper facial skeleton and lower facial skeleton (mandible).

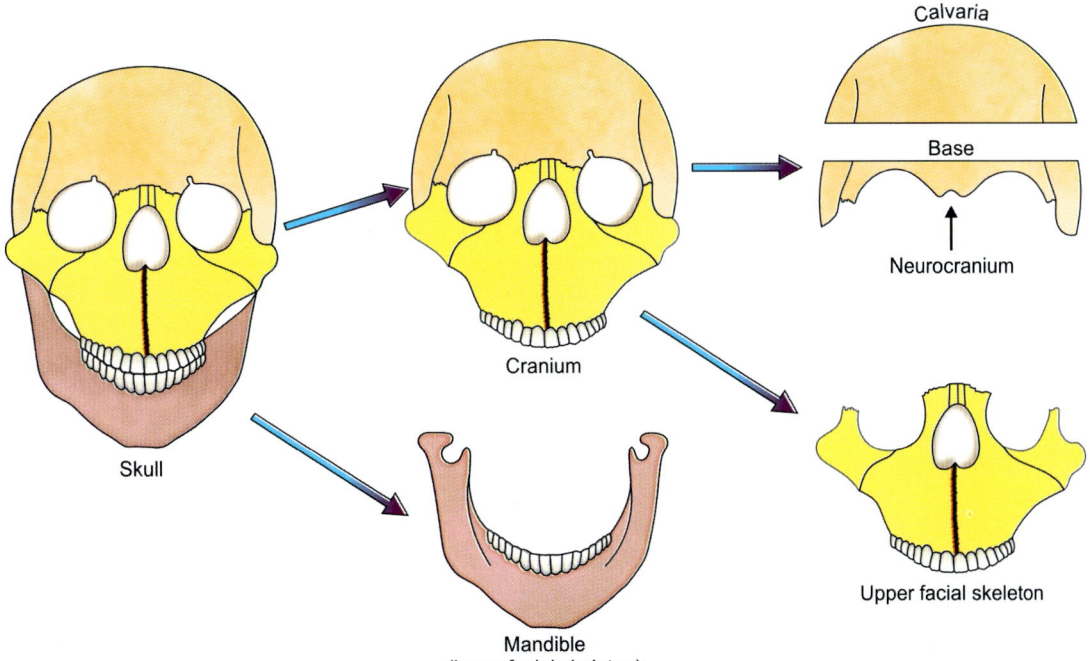

**Fig. 2.1:** Subdivisions of skull

## NEUROCRANIUM

The bones which constitute the neurocranium can be classified as:

### A. Paired bones
These include:
  a. Parietal bones.
  b. Temporal bones.

### B. Unpaired bones
These include:
  a. Frontal bone.
  b. Occipital bone.
  c. Sphenoid.
  d. Ethmoid.

## FACIAL SKELETON (VISCEROCRANIUM OR SPLANCHNOCRANIUM)

It is composed of following bones:

### A. Paired bones
These include:
  a. Maxillae.
  b. Zygomatic bones.
  c. Nasal bones.
  d. Lacrimal bones.
  e. Palatine bones.
  f. Inferior conchae.

### B. Unpaired bones
These include:
  a. Mandible.
  b. Vomer.

## ANATOMICAL POSITION OF SKULL (Fig. 2.2)

Skull can be kept in normal anatomical position by Reid's baseline or Frankfurt's horizontal plane.

### A. Reid's baseline
It is a horizontal line formed by the joining of infraorbital margin with the centre of the external acoustic meatus.

### B. Frankfurt's horizontal plane
It is marked by the horizontal line joining the infraorbital margin with the upper margin of the external acoustic meatus.

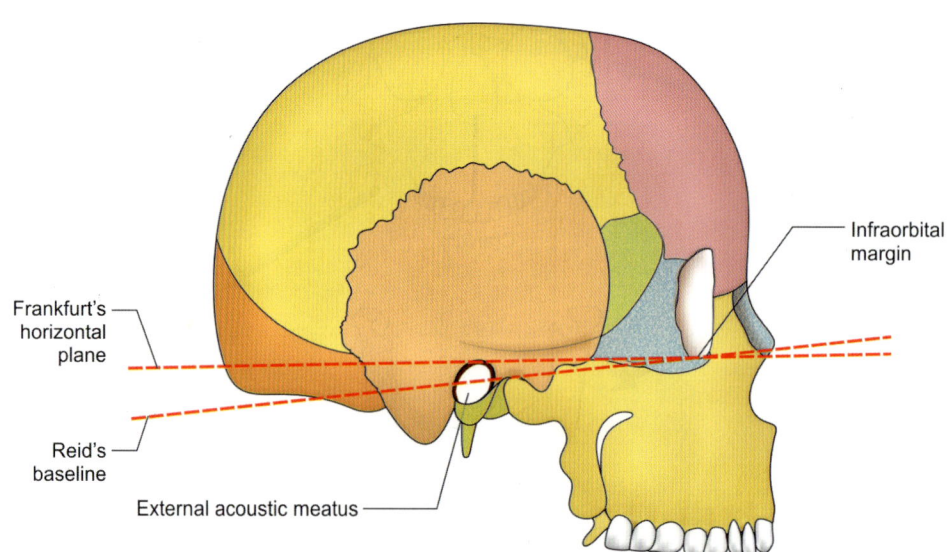

**Fig. 2.2:** Skull in relation to horizontal planes

**Note:** *Remember that Reid's starts with 'R' which also stands for 'Round' opening of external acoustic meatus, thus Reid's baseline passes through the rounded external acoustic meatus. On the other hand 'Frankfurt' starts with 'F' which also stands for 'Fly' and anything that has to fly has to be above, therefore, Frankfurt's horizontal plane passes above the external acoustic meatus.*

## APPLIED ANATOMY

Clinically the entire front of skull is considered to be facial skeleton. It is further divided into following three parts (Fig. 2.3):

### I. Upper facial skeleton

1. It forms the skeleton of forehead.
2. It is comprised of frontal bone.

### II. Lower facial skeleton

1. It forms the skeleton of the lower jaw.
2. It is comprised of mandible.

### III. Middle facial skeleton

It is the complex middle 3rd of the facial skeleton. The region is of great clinical importance because the multiple bones constituting it are frequently involved in fractures.

### A. Boundaries

   *a. Upper:* Transverse line passing through frontozygomatic, frontomaxillary and frontonasal sutures.

   *b. Lower:* Incisal edge and occlusal plane.

   *c. Posterior:* Spheno-ethmoidal junction.

### B. Bones involved in the fractures of middle 3rd of the facial skeleton are as follows:

1. Maxillae.
2. Palatine bones.
3. Zygomatic bones.
4. Zygomatic processes of temporal bones.
5. Nasal bones.
6. Lacrimal bones.
7. Vomer.
8. Ethmoid.
9. Pterygoid processes of sphenoid.

### C. Subdivisions (Fig. 2.4)

The middle 3rd facial skeleton can be divided into:

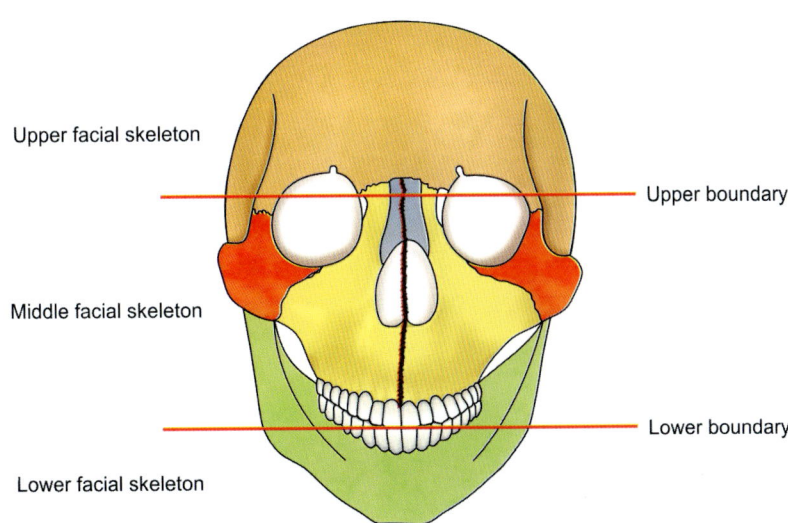

**Fig. 2.3:** Subdivisions of facial skeleton

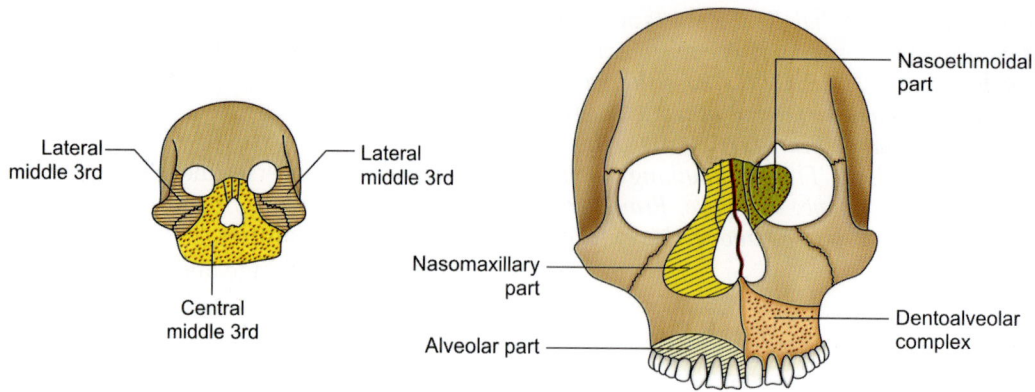

**Fig. 2.4:** Clinical subdivisions of middle 3rd of facial skeleton

a. **Lateral middle 3rd** also called zygomatico-maxillary part.

b. **Central middle 3rd,** which can be further subdivided into:

 i. Alveolar part.
 ii. Dentoalveolar complex.
 iii. Nasomaxillary part.
 iv. Nasoethmoidal part.

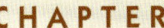

# CHAPTER

# 3

# Exterior of the Skull

Different views of skull are considered from the description point of view. These are as follows:

  **I. Norma verticalis:** This is superior view.
 **II. Norma occipitalis:** This is posterior view.
**III. Norma frontalis:** This is anterior view.
 **IV. Norma lateralis:** This is lateral (side) view.
  **V. Norma basalis:** This is inferior view.

## I. NORMA VERTICALIS

### Definition

Observation of skull from superior aspect is called norma verticalis.

### Shape

Norma verticalis view of skull appears ovoid in shape. It is relatively wider posteriorly.

### Bones

The following bones contribute to the norma verticalis:

1. *Frontal bone (frontal squama)*: It lies anteriorly.
2. *Occipital bone (squamous part)*: It lies posteriorly.
3. *Parietal bones (paired)*: These lie on each side of midline.

## Junctions of Bones (sutures)

1. Sutures are the immovable joints of skull which are fibrous in nature.

2. In norma verticalis following sutures can be seen:

   i. *Coronal suture*: It is between frontal and parietal bones.

  ii. *Sagittal suture:* It is between the two parietal bones.

 iii. *Lambdoid suture:* It is between occipital and two parietal bones.

## Features (Fig. 3.1)

### a. Vertex

It is the highest point on sagittal suture.

### b. Vault

It is the arched roof of skull.

### c. Bregma

1. It is situated at the intersection between coronal and sagittal sutures.

2. Bregma is the site of a membranous gap in the foetal skull. This gap is known as *anterior fontanelle*.

3. Anterior fontanelle closes by 18 months.

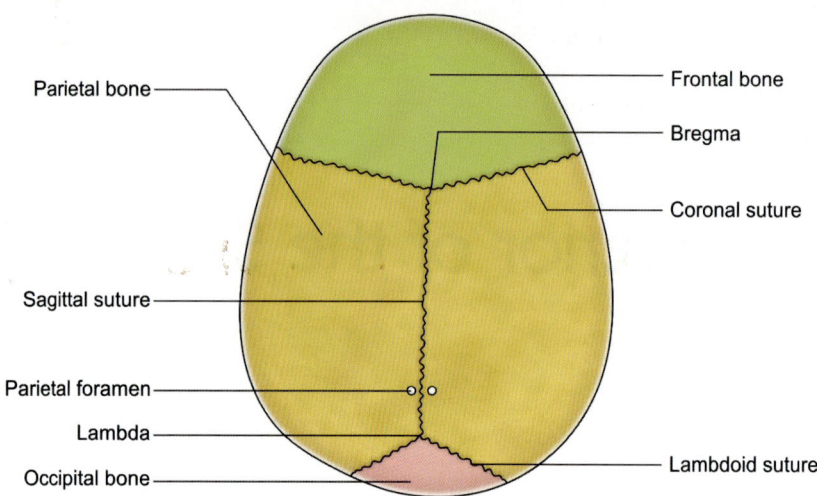

**Fig. 3.1:** The skull: Norma verticalis

### d. Lambda

1. It is situated at the intersection of sagittal and lambdoid sutures.
2. In foetal skull there is a membranous gap at the site of lambda. This gap is known as *posterior fontanelle*.
3. Posterior fontanelle closes by 2–3 months.

### e. Parietal foramen

It pierces the parietal bone on each side of midline about 3.5 cm in front of lambda. *Emissary vein* passes through it.

### f. Obelion

It is the region on the sagittal suture between two parietal foramina.

### g. Parietal eminence

It is the area of maximum convexity of the parietal bone.

### h. Temporal lines

1. There are two temporal lines on each side:
   i. *Superior temporal line.*
   ii. *Inferior temporal line.*
2. Both the temporal lines start as single line from the zygomatic process of frontal bone.

3. The two lines arch backwards and upwards and cross the frontal bone, coronal suture and parietal bone.
4. Superior temporal line fades out in the posterior part of parietal bone.
5. *Epicranial aponeurosis* and temporal fascia are attached to superior temporal line.
6. Inferior temporal line marks the upper limit of the origin of *temporalis muscle.*

### Applied anatomy

1. Fontanelles serve two important purposes:
   i. These allow moulding during birth.
   ii. These allow the brain to grow.
2. The presence of *anterior fontanelle* is both clinically and therapeutically very significant.
   i. A buldge indicates increased intracranial tension (*e.g. in case of brain tumour*).
   ii. An abnormal depression indicates excessive loss of fluid (*e.g. in case of bleeding and dehydration*).
   iii. *Diagnostic* and *therapeutic punctures* could be carried out through anterior fontanelle.

iv. *Ultrasonography* of brain in infants is performed through anterior fontanelle.

3. The osseous closure of the anterior fontanelle is an important milestone in the normal development of a child.

4. Soft and pliable bones of neonate can withstand considerable amount of compression and moulding, a fact clinically important during child birth.

5. In neonates the flat bones of the vault are very soft and, therefore, a depressed fracture is like a dimple (*pond fracture*).

6. In adult there is some amount of elasticity in flat vault bones which often prevents fractures in cases of minor trauma. But if the trauma force exceeds the minimal elasticity, fractures are bound to occur.

7. In adult a *depressed fracture* always shows an irregular line of fracture at the periphery of depressed area.

8. Almost invariably all fractures of the vault of skull in children are associated with the rupture of the dura mater.

9. When skull is compressed between two hard surfaces an axial shortening takes place along the line of the force and an axial lengthening takes place at right angle to it. This results in fracture of distant poles of the skull far from the actual site of application of force (Fig. 3.2).

10. *Fracture* of the skull is usually due to direct blow. A forceful hit on the forehead may cause linear fracture of vertex (Fig. 3.3).

11. Cranium is clinically important because it reflects the size of the brain. *Macrocephaly* (enlargement of head) can be due to hydrocephalus. *Microcephaly* may be hereditary or due to maldevelopment of brain.

12. Because of the lack of regenerating capacity of the flat bones of the vault, a gap in it should be filled with *tantalum* or *titanium*.

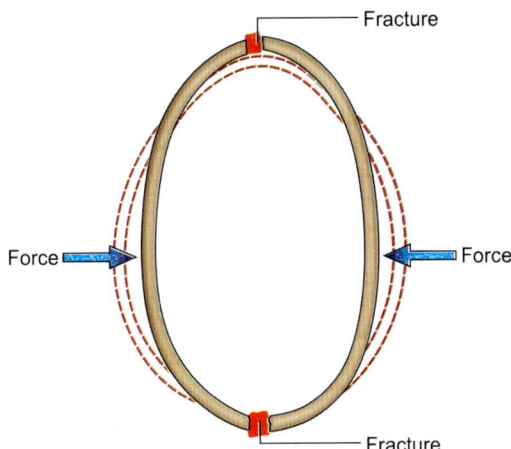

**Fig. 3.2:** Axial deformity of skull due to compression

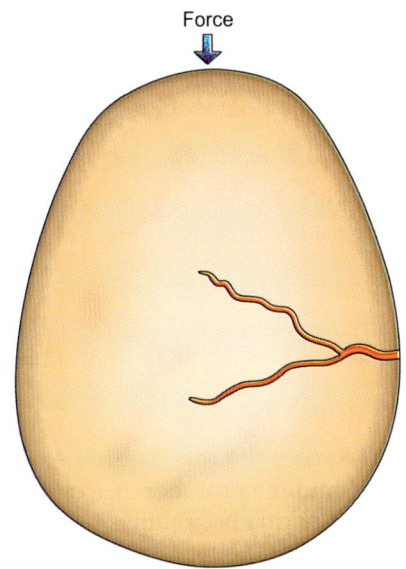

**Fig. 3.3:** Linear fracture of vertex

## II. NORMA OCCIPITALIS

### Definition

When the skull is observed from posterior aspect, it is known as norma occipitalis.

## Shape

Norma occipitalis is convex upwards and flat below.

## Bones

Following bones contribute to the norma occipitalis.

1. *Parietal bones* (paired).
2. Squamous part of *occipital bone* (unpaired).
3. Mastoid parts of *temporal bones* (paired).

## Sutures

### a. Posterior part of sagittal suture

### b. Lambdoid suture

1. It is between the two parietal bones and the occipital bone.
2. The lower end of lambdoid suture meets with the mastoid portion of temporal bone at a point which forms the junction of *occipitomastoid* and *parietomastoid* *sutures*.

### c. Occipitomastoid suture

It is situated between the occipital bone and the mastoid part of the temporal bone.

### d. Parietomastoid suture

It is situated between the parietal bone and the mastoid part of the temporal bone.

## Features (Fig. 3.4)

### a. External occipital protuberance

1. It is a midline protuberance on the lower part of norma occipitalis.
2. It marks the junction of head and neck posteriorly.
3. *Inion* is the most prominent point of external occipital protuberance.
4. *Trapezius* originates from the upper part of external occipital protuberance.
5. *Ligamentum nuchae* is attached to the lower part of this protuberance.

### b. Superior nuchal lines

1. These are curved ridges passing laterally from the external occipital protuberance.

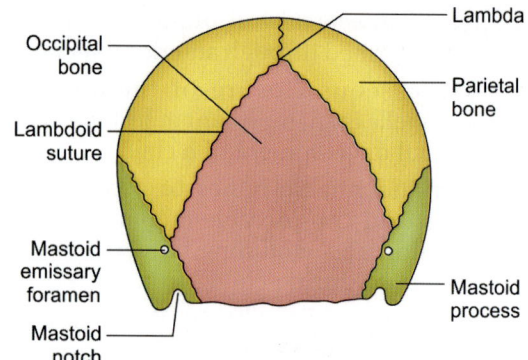

**Fig. 3.4:** The skull: Norma occipitalis

2. These form junction of head and neck posteriorly.
3. *Trapezius* originates from the medial 1/3rd of superior nuchal line.
4. *Sternocleidomastoid* is inserted on the lateral part of superior nuchal line.
5. *Splenius capitis* is also inserted on the lateral part of this line below the attachment of sternomastoid.

### c. Highest nuchal lines

1. These are situated about a 'cm' above the superior nuchal lines.
2. *Epicranial aponeurosis* is attached to their medial parts.
3. *Occipital belly of occipitofrontalis* originates on each side from its lateral 2/3rd.

### d. Mastoid foramen

1. It is located near the occipitomastoid suture.
2. It opens internally into the sigmoid sulcus.
3. Following structures transverse through it:
   i. *Meningeal branch of occipital artery.*
   ii. *Emissary vein.*

### e. Occipital point

1. It is situated in the midline a little above the inion.
2. It is farthest from glabella.

## Applied anatomy

1. *Craniostenosis* is the condition in which there is premature closure of the cranial sutures. When lambdoid and coronal sutures are involved, skull grows vertically leading to *tower skull.*

2. The squamous part of the occipital bone is prone to both *fissured and depressed fractures.*

3. A crack the inner table of squamous part of occipital bone may damage the large diploeic vein and produce small *epidural haematoma.*

4. Almost invariably fractures of the occipital squama in children are associated with *rupture of the dura mater.*

5. A gap in the occipital squama is usually filled with *tantalum or titanium* due to lack of regeneration in this part whose periosteum is devoid of cambium layer.

6. Inner table of cranial vault bones (including squamous part of occipital bone) is more brittle than the outer table, therefore, fractures are more extensive in the inner table.

## III. NORMA FRONTALIS

### Definition

When the skull is observed from the anterior aspect it is known as norma frontalis.

### Shape

It is oval in shape being wider above than below.

### Bones

Major bones contributing to the surface features of norma frontalis (excluding bones contributing to deeper orbits, nasal cavity and oral cavity) are as follows:

1. *Frontal bone* (unpaired).
2. *Maxillae* (paired).
3. *Nasal bones* (paired).
4. *Zygomatic bones* (paired).
5. *Mandible ethmoid* (unpaired).

## Junctions of Bones (Sutures)

a. Junction between zygomatic process of frontal bone and frontal process of zygomatic bone is called *frontozygomatic suture.* It is observed along the lateral margin of orbital opening.

b. Junction between nasal part of frontal bone and frontal process of maxilla (*fronto-maxillary suture*) is observed along the medial margin of orbital opening in its upper part.

c. Junction between nasal part of frontal bone and nasal bones are called *frontonasal sutures.*

d. Junction between two nasal bones is a midline suture just above the anterior nasal aperture. This is called *internasal suture.*

e. Junction between maxilla and zygomatic bone (*zygomaticomaxillary suture*) is an oblique suture extending downwards and laterally from the lower border of each orbital opening.

f. Junction between two maxillae is called *intermaxillary suture.* It is a midline suture just below the anterior nasal aperture.

**Note:** *Intermaxillary suture is also observed in hard palate between palatine processes of two maxillae.*

### Features (Fig. 3.5)

#### A. Three large apertures

One anterior nasal aperture and two orbital openings form the most striking feature of the norma frontalis.

#### a. Anterior nasal aperture

1. It is a midline aperture.
2. It is piriform in shape and wider below than above.
3. Its upper boundary is formed by lower borders of nasal bones.
4. Its lateral and inferior boundaries are contributed by nasal notches of two maxillae.

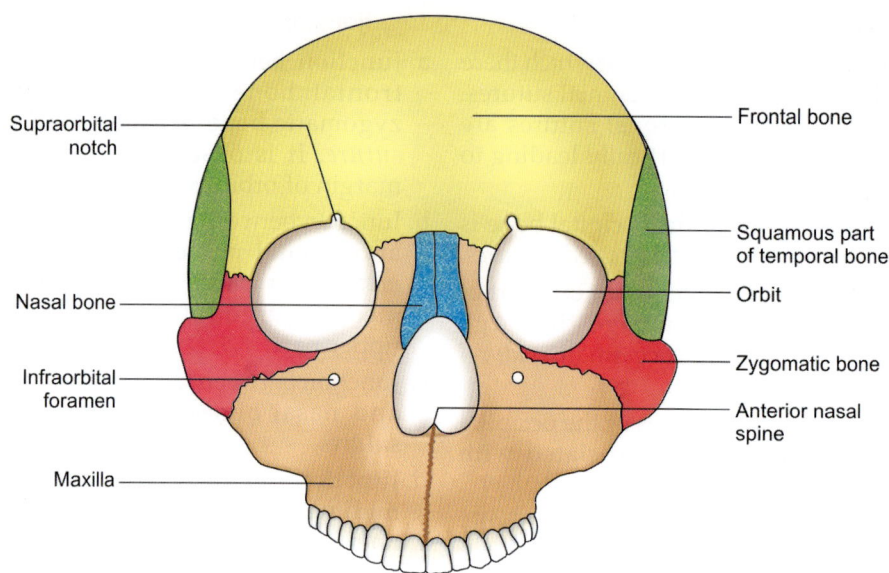

**Fig. 3.5:** The skull: Norma frontalis

5. *Anterior nasal spine* is a sharp projection at the lower margin of nasal aperture, in the midline.
6. *Rhinion* is the lower end of internasal suture.
7. A notch at the inferior border of nasal bone is meant for passage of *external nasal nerve*.
8. Margins of aperture give attachments to the *nasal cartilages*.

### b. Orbital openings

Each is present above and lateral to the anterior nasal aperture. It is quadrangular in shape and possesses four margins (*supraorbital, infraorbital, lateral* and *medial*).

  i. *Supraorbital margin*
1. It is formed by frontal bone.
2. *Supraorbital notch (or foramen)* is situated at the junction of medial 1/3rd (rounded) and lateral 2/3rds (sharp) of supraorbital margin.
3. Supraorbital notch transmits *supraorbital nerve and artery and a communicating vein between angular and superior ophthalmic veins*.

  ii. *Infraorbital margin*

It is formed by *maxilla* medially and *zygomatic bone* laterally.

  iii. *Lateral orbital margin*

It is formed by the *frontal process* of zygomatic bone below and the *zygomatic process of frontal bone* above.

  iv. *Medial orbital margin*

It is formed by the *frontal bone* above and the *lacrimal crest of frontal process of maxilla below*.

### B. Frontal region

### a. Superciliary arch

It is curved elevation above the medial part of the supraorbital margin.

### b. Glabella

It is median elevation between two superciliary arches.

### c. Nasion

It is the junction of internasal and frontonasal sutures.

**d. Frontal eminence (frontal tuber)**

It is rounded elevation above each superciliary arch.

## C. Maxillae

Each maxilla shows following features:

**a. Infraorbital foramen**

1. It is situated about 1 cm below the infraorbital margin.
2. *Infraorbital nerve and vessels* pass through infraorbital foramen.

**b. Incisive fossa**

It is situated above the incisor teeth.

**c. Canine eminence**

It is produced by the root of canine tooth.

**d. Canine fossa**

It is situated just lateral to canine eminence.

**e. Frontal process**

It is sandwiched between nasal bone and lacrimal bone.

**f. Zygomatic process**

It articulates with the zygomatic bone.

**g. Alveolar process**

It bears the sockets for the upper teeth.

## D. Zygomatic bones

1. Each bone is situated below and lateral to the orbital opening.
2. It is marked by a foramen called *zygomaticofacial foramen*.
3. *Zygomaticofacial nerve* traverses the zygomaticofacial foramen.

## E. Mandible

It forms the lower facial skeleton. For details of the features please consult the description of individual bone.

## Attachments (Fig. 3.6)

A. Nasal bone: *Procerus*

B. Superciliary arch: *Corrugator supercilii*

C. Frontal process of maxilla.

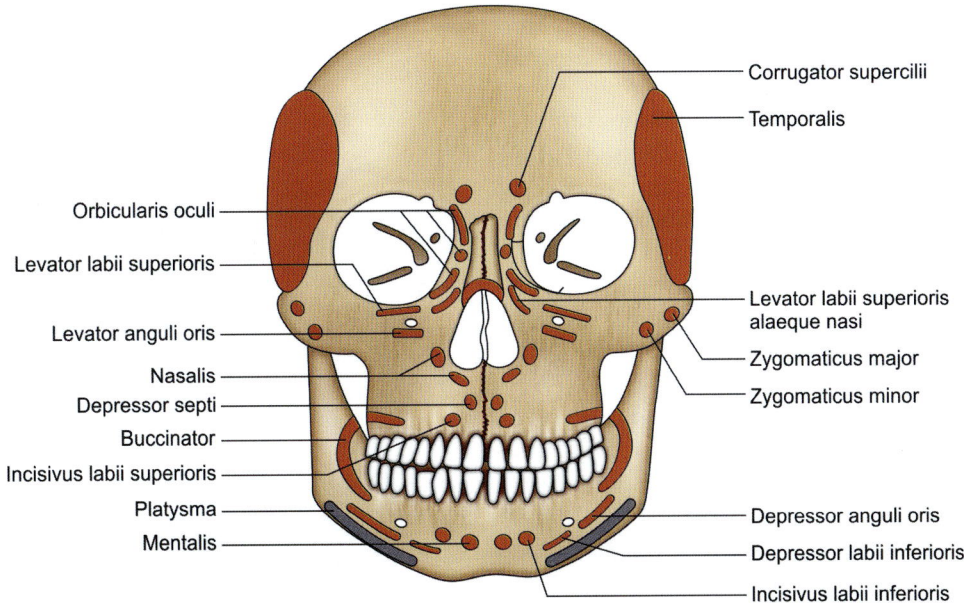

**Fig. 3.6:** Attachments on skull: Norma frontalis

1. *Orbital part of orbicularis oculi* (it is also attached to nasal part of frontal bone).
2. *Medial palpebral ligament.*
3. *Levator babii superioris alaeque nasi.*

D. Between infraorbital margin and infraorbital foramen: *Levator labii superioris.*

E. Below the infraorbital foramen (to canine fossa): *Levator anguli oris.*

F. Zygomatic bone just below the zygomaticofacial foramen: *Zygomaticus minor.*

G. Lateral to zygomaticus minor: *Zygomaticus major.*

H. Adjacent to nasal notch: *Nasalis* (transverse part above and alar part below).

I. Incisive fossa.

Medially: *Depressor septi*

Laterally: *Incisivus labii superioris.*

J. Alveolar process of maxilla opposite to molar teeth: *Buccinator.*

K. Mandible: Please consult the description of individual bone.

## Applied anatomy

1. In about 8% of adult skulls a remnant of lower part of the suture between two halves of frontal bone (*metopic suture*) may persist. This suture is some times confused for a fracture in radiograph.
2. Superciliary arches are elevated ridges from the surface of bone and any injury in this region will cause laceration of skin and severe bleeding.
3. Compression of supraorbital nerves causes nerve pain. This fact may be used by anaesthetists to determine the depth of anaesthesia.
4. If the fracture of the frontal bone involves inner table forming the roof of the frontal sinus, then the air may enter the cranial cavity (*aerocele*) causing meningitis or brain abscess.
5. An impact on the nose directed in the anteroposterior plane will cause a depression of the nasal bridge due to fracture of nasal bones, frontal processes of maxillae and septal cartilage.

6. A force on the nasal bridge directed from the lateral aspect will result in a deviation of the nasal bridge to opposite side.
7. Traumatic alteration in the shape of nose because of fractures of nasal bones is of great clinical importance due to cosmetic reasons specially in young females.
8. A severe impact on the nasal bridge may involve frontal processes of maxillae.
9. Mid-facial skeleton is commonly involved in facial injuries. It includes maxillae, zygomatic bones, nasal bones and most of the bones which form nasal cavity.
10. Mid-facial skeleton receives adequate blood supply from periosteal arteries and, therefore, all the fragments of fractured bone retain a periosteal blood supply.
11. Fractures of maxillae and zygomatic bones show a constant pattern. Le Fort has classified such fractures into three types (Fig. 3.7):

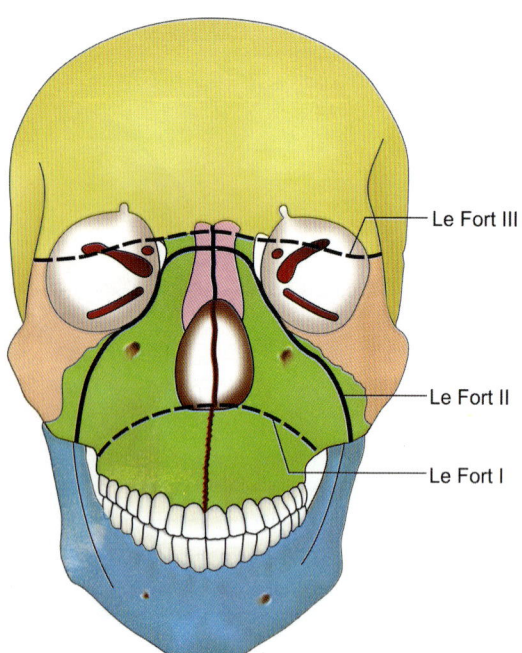

Le Fort III

Le Fort II

Le Fort I

**Fig. 3.7:** Common fractures of maxillae and other bones of skull

i. *Le Fort I fracture (Guerin's fracture):* It shows fractures of lower 3rd of nasal septum, maxillae and lower 3rd of pterygoid plates.

ii. *Le Fort II fracture:* It includes fractures of nasal bones, frontal processes of maxillae, lacrimal bones, ethmoid, vomer and pterygoid plates.

iii. *Le Fort III fracture:* In this fracture facial skeleton is separated from skull base. It involves upper parts of nasal bones, frontal processes of maxillae, ethmoid, lesser wings of sphenoid and roots of pterygoid plates.

12. Zygomatic bone is very commonly involved in cases of fractures of middle 3rd of face. Fracture of the frontal process of the zygomatic bone may occur in conjuction with a comminuted fracture of the orbital rim and frontal bone.

13. Any of the four margins of the orbit may fracture as isolated fracture or in combination.

**Note:** *For applied anatomy of mandible and other bones of norma frontalis, discussion on individual bone may be consulted.*

## IV. NORMA LATERALIS

### Definition

When skull is observed from side, it constitutes norma lateralis.

### Bones

Following bones can be visualized in this view:
1. *Frontal*
2. *Parietal*
3. *Occipital*
4. *Nasal*
5. *Zygomatic*
6. *Temporal*
7. *Sphenoid*
8. *Maxilla*

### Features and attachments (Fig. 3.8)

#### A. Temporal lines

There are two temporal lines, superior and inferior.

##### a. Superior temporal line

1. It commences at frontal process of zygomatic bone.
2. It arches upwards and backwards across parietal bone.

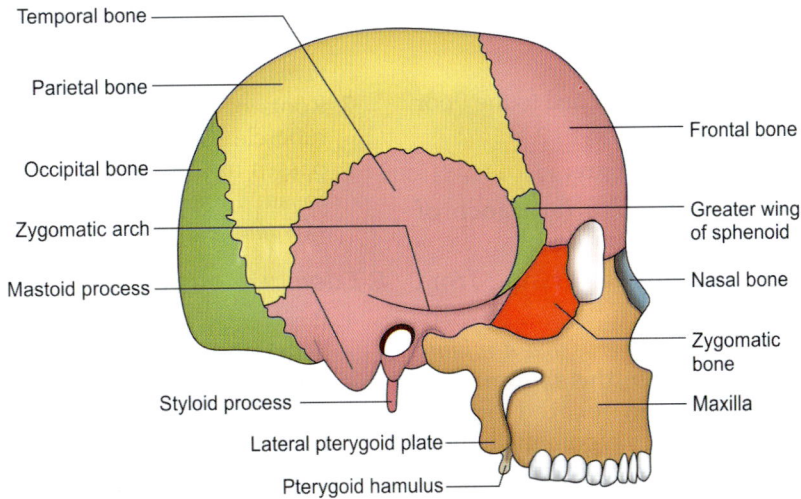

**Fig. 3.8:** The skull: Norma lateralis

3. It fades away on temporal bone.

4. *Temporal fasia* is attached to it.

### b. Inferior temporal line

1. It commences at the same point.

2. It runs inferior and parallel to the superior temporal line.

3. Posteriorly it curves downwards and forwards on the temporal bone to continue with supramastoid crest.

4. It limits the attachment of *temporalis muscle.*

## B. Temporal fossa

### i. Boundaries

1. Anteriorly: *Zygomatic bone.*

2. Superiorly: *Superior temporal line.*

3. Posteriorly: *Superior temporal line.*
                   *Supramastoid crest.*

4. Inferiorly: *Zygomatic arch.*

### ii. Anterior wall of the fossa is formed by:

1. *Temporal surface of zygomatic bone*

2. *Greater wing of sphenoid*

3. *Frontal bone*

### iii. Its floor is formed by following bones:

1. *Frontal*

2. *Parietal*

3. *Temporal*

4. *Greater wing of sphenoid.*

### iv. Temporalis muscle is attached to the floor and inferior temporal line.

### v. Other contents of fossa are:

1. *Middle temporal artery* (a branch of superficial temporal artery).

2. *Deep temporal arteries* arising from maxillary artery.

3. *Zygomaticotemporal nerve and a minute artery* appears from the zygomatico-temporal foramen located on the temporal surface of zygomatic bone.

4. *Deep temporal nerves* arising from mandibular nerve.

## C. Pterion

1. It is a circular area in the anterior part of temporal fossa which encloses four bones, *frontal, parietal, sphenoid* and *temporal.* These four bones form an 'H' shaped suture.

2. It is located 4 cm above the zygomatic arch and 3.5 cm behind the fronto-zygomatic suture.

3. *Middle meningeal vein, anterior branch of middle meningeal artery* and *stem of the lateral sulcus of brain* lie deep to pterion.

## D. Zygomatic arch

1. It is formed by the *temporal process of zygomatic bone* and *zygomatic process of temporal bone.*

2. It has two surfaces (outer and inner) and two borders (upper and lower).

3. Its outer surface is subcutaneous and crossed by following structures from posterior to anterior:

   i. *Auriculotemporal nerve.*

   ii. *Superficial temporal vein.*

   iii. *Superficial temporal artery.*

4. *Masseter* originates from its inner surface and lower border.

5. *Temporal fascia* is attached to its upper border.

6. Posterior end of lower border is marked by *tubercle of root of zygoma.* To this is attached *lateral ligament of temporo-mandibular joint.*

7. Roots of zygomatic arch diverge from tubercle. Anterior root (*articular tubercle*) passes medially in front of mandibular fossa. Posterior root continues with *supramastoid crest.*

## E. External acoustic meatus

1. It is located behind the mandibular fossa below the posterior root of zygoma.

2. Its anterior wall, floor and lower part of posterior wall is formed by the tympanic part while its roof and upper part of posterior wall is contributed by squamous part of temporal bone.

3. Margins of the meatus give attachment to *cartilaginous part of external acoustic meatus.*

### F. MacEwen's triangle (suprameatal triangle)

1. It is situated posterosuperior to external acoustic meatus.
2. *Spine of Henle (suprameatal spine)* may be present at the anteroinferior part of triangle.
3. Mastoid antrum is situated about 12.5 mm deep to suprameatal triangle.

### g. Mastoid process

1. It is a downward projection from the mastoid part of temporal bone.
2. It is present below and behind the external acoustic meatus.
3. The muscles attached to it from anterior to posterior are:
   i. *Sternocleidomastoid.*
   ii. *Splenius capitis.*
   iii. *Longissimus capitis.*
4. *Posterior belly of digastric* originates from its medial aspect (*digastric notch*).

### H. Styloid process

1. It is a slender, elongated projection below the external acoustic meatus and in front of mastoid process.
2. It provides attachments to following five structures:
   i. Anteriorly: *Styloglossus muscle.*
   ii. Posteriorly: *Stylohyoid muscle.*
   iii. Medially: *Stylopharyngeus muscle.*
   iv. Laterally: *Stylomandibular ligament.*
   v. On the tip: *Stylohyoid ligament.*

### i. Infratemporal fossa

It is an irregular space below the zygomatic arch.

**a. Boundaries**

Anterior : Posterior surface of body of maxilla.

Medial – Lateral pterygoid plate and pyramidal process of palatine bone.

Lateral – Ramus of mandible

Roof – Infratemporal surface of greater wing of sphenoid.

**b. Contents**
   i. *Muscles*
      1. *Lateral and medial pterygoids.*
      2. *Temporalis.*
   ii. *Arteries*
      1. *Maxillary artery* (Ist and 2nd parts) with its branches.
      2. *Posterior superior alveolar branch* of 3rd part of maxillary artery.
   iii. *Veins*
      1. *Maxillary vein.*
      2. *Pterygoid venous plexus.*
      3. *Posterior superior alveolar vein.*
   iv. *Nerves*
      1. *Mandibular nerve and its branches.*
      2. *Chorda tympani.*
      3. *Maxillary nerve.*
      4. *Posterior superior alveolar nerve.*

**c. Anterior wall** of the fossa shows two to three perforations for the *posterior superior alveolar nerve and vessels.*

**d.** Junction of anterior and medial walls is marked by a fissure (**pterygomaxillary fissure**) through which it communicates with pterygopalatine fossa.

**e.** The junction of roof and anterior wall is marked by **lateral part of inferior orbital fissure.**

**f.** *Foramen ovale* and *foramen supinosum* are present in the **roof of the fossa.**

**g. Lateral part of fossa** communicates with temporal fossa through a gap between zygomatic arch and side of skull.

### J. Pterygomaxillary fissure

1. It is a gap which leads into pterygo-palatine fossa.

2. *Boundaries*

Anterior: Maxilla.

Posterior: Pterygoid process.

3. *Maxillary artery* enters the pterygo-palatine fossa through pterygomaxillary fissure.

4. *Maxillary nerve* courses forwards through it from pterygopalatine fossa to enter the orbit through inferior orbital fissure.

## K. Pterygopalatine fossa

### a. Boundaries

Anterior: Posterior surface of *maxilla.*

Posterior: 1. *Pterygoid process.*

　　　　　2. *Greater wing of sphenoid.*

Medial: Perpendicular plate of *palatine bone.*

Floor: Fusion of anterior and posterior walls.

### b. Communications

The pterygopalatine fossa communicates with,

1. The orbit, through the inferior orbital fissure.

2. The middle cranial fossa, through foramen rotundum.

3. The infratemporal fossa, through pterygomaxillary fissure.

4. The nasal cavity, through palatovaginal canal and sphenopalatine foramen.

5. The foramen lacerum, through pterygoid canal.

### c. Contents

1. *Third part of maxillary artery and its branches.*

2. *Maxillary nerve with its branches.*

3. *Pterygopalatine ganglion and its branches.*

## Applied anatomy

1. *Spine of Henle* is an important surgical landmark for surgery on mastoid antrum.

2. *Pterion* is very important clinically because the anterior branch of middle meningeal artery and accompanying vein lie on its internal aspect and are vulnerable to tearing if there are fractures of bone forming this region.

3. If the meningeal vessels in the region of pterion are damaged, an *extradural haematoma* is formed. Such haematoma may exert pressure on the cerebral cortex.

4. Decompression of brain in cases of extradural haematoma in the region of pterion can be done by the method of *trephining* (burr hole) at this site.

5. Temporal fascia is commonly used for making *tympanic membrane graft* during surgery for repair of ear drum.

6. Deep temporal vessels and nerves along with the tendon of temporalis muscle, transverse the gap deep to zygomatic arch whose fracture can involve these structures.

7. An *elongated styloid process* usually needs surgical correction because it leads to multiple complications in the neck.

8. An *oblique line drawn from the frontozygomatic suture to the pterion* corresponds with inferior surface of frontal lobe. This surface landmark is of great neurosurgical importance.

9. In radiographs of skull, the *diploic canals* containing the diploic veins may be mistaken for the fractures of skull.

10. *Calvaria* is very thin in the region of temporal fossa and, therefore, is likely to get fractured because of hard blows to the head.

11. In *depressed fractures*, the inner table of calvaria is often more extensively fractured than the outer table.

12. *Zygomatic fracture* is very common in facial injuries due to its prominent position.

13. *Fracture of skull* is usually due to direct blows. A forceful hit on the forehead causes linear fractures of both vertex and base (Fig. 3.9).

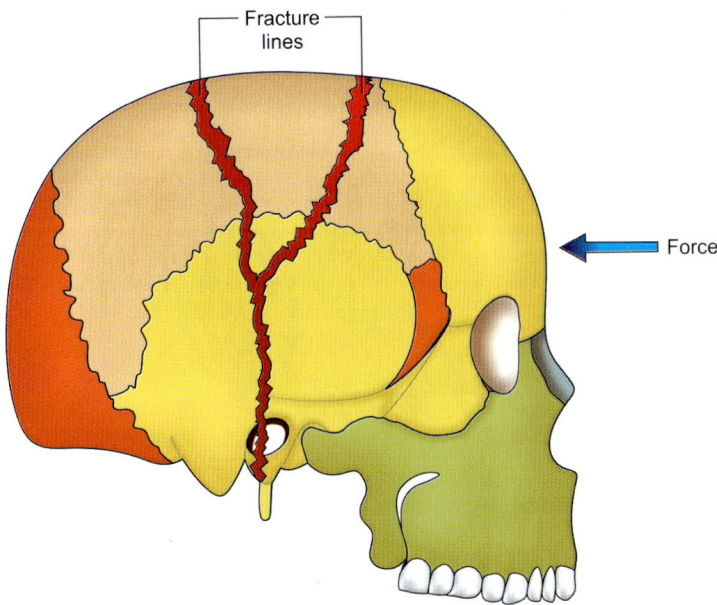

**Fig. 3.9:** Fracture of skull due to blow on the forehead

14. Junctions of frontal and temporal processes of zygomatic bone form surgically important landmark in the treatment of *maxillofacial injuries.*

15. The periosteum and attachment of strong temporal fascia limit the *displacement of zygomatic bone* following injuries.

16. In *depressed fracture* of zygomatico-maxillary complex the maxilla is greatly damaged and there is displacement of zygomatic bone without its fracture (Fig. 3.10).

17. If *fracture of zygomatic arch* is associated with separation from temporal fascia, then there occurs a downward displacement of arch.

18. The weakest point of zygomatic arch is its middle, just behind the temporo-zygomatic suture. This point is the commonest to fracture in cases of injuries to the arch.

19. *Frontozygomatic suture,* the *zygomatic prominence, the zygomatic buttress* and *1st molar tooth lie in the same vertical line.* In majority of zygomatic-complex (zygomatic bone + adjacent bones like maxilla and zygomatic process of temporal) fracture, the zygomatic bone rotates along this axis (Fig. 3.11).

## V. NORMA BASALIS

### Definition

Observation of cranium (skull without mandible) from inferior aspect is called norma basalis.

### Boundaries

Anterior: *Incisor teeth.*

Posterior: *Superior nuchal line.*

Lateral (side):

1. *Rest of teeth.*
2. *Zygomatic arch.*
3. *Posterior root of zygoma.*
4. *Mastoid process.*

### Subdivisions

For the sake of convenience, norma basalis is divided into anterior, middle and posterior

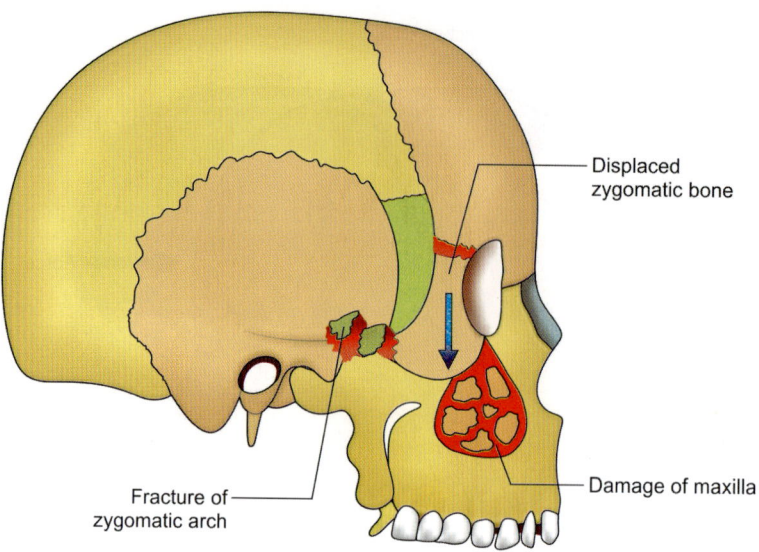

**Fig. 3.10:** Depressed fracture of zygomatico-maxillary complex

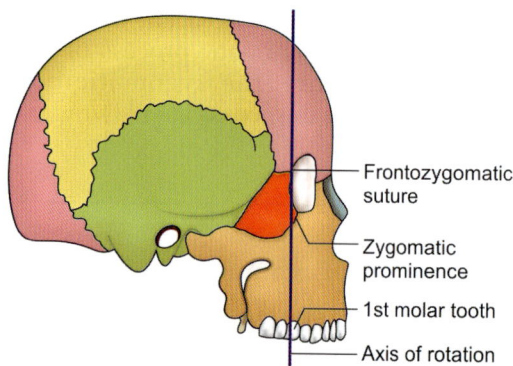

**Fig. 3.11:** Axis of rotation of zygomatic bone in zygomatic complex fracture

parts. Hard palate and alveolar arch are included in the anterior part. An imaginary horizontal line passing through the anterior margin of foramen magnum separates the posterior part from the middle part of norma basalis.

## Features and attachments (Figs 3.12 and 3.13)

### A. Anterior part of norma basalis

#### a. Posterior border of hard palate

1. It forms the junction of anterior and middle parts of norma basalis.
2. *Posterior nasal spine* is a spinous projection from its middle in the median plane.
3. *Musculus uvulae* is attached to posterior nasal spine.

#### b. Alveolar arch

1. It possesses *sockets for the roots of upper teeth.*
2. Number of sockets depends upon number of roots. There is single socket for each of the incisors, canines and premolars. There are three sockets for each of the upper molars.

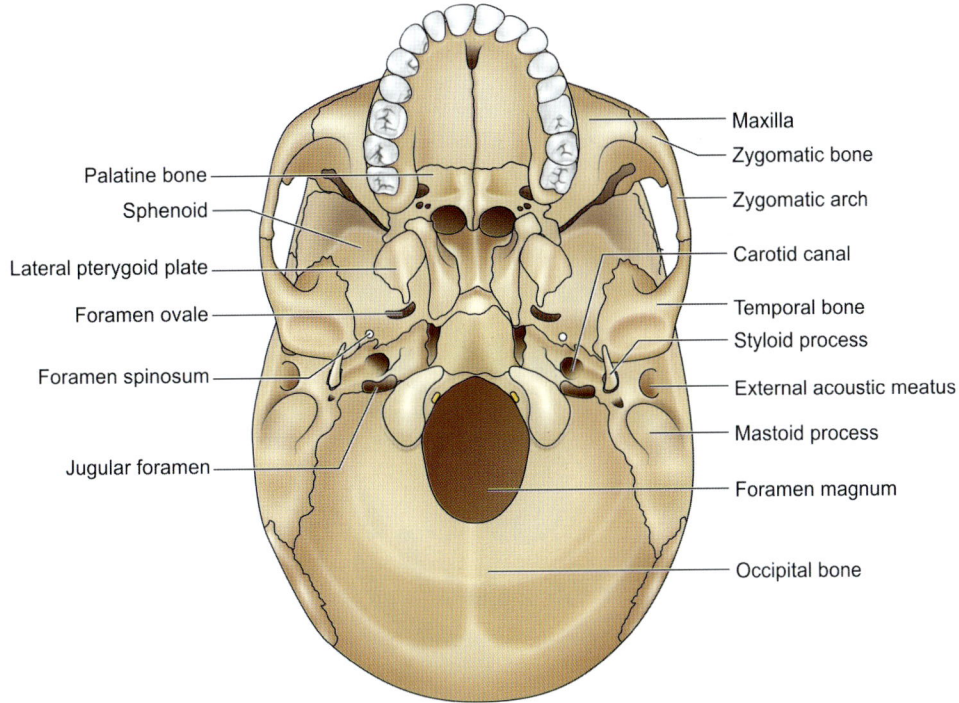

Palatine bone

Sphenoid

Lateral pterygoid plate

Foramen ovale

Foramen spinosum

Jugular foramen

Maxilla

Zygomatic bone

Zygomatic arch

Carotid canal

Temporal bone

Styloid process

External acoustic meatus

Mastoid process

Foramen magnum

Occipital bone

**Fig. 3.12:** The skull: Norma basalis

### c. Bones contributing to hard palate

1. *Palatine processes* of *two maxillae* contribute to the anterior 2/3rd of the hard palate.
2. Posterior 1/3rd of the hard palate is formed by the *horizontal plates* of *palatine bones.*
3. Bony palate is marked by several depressions produced by *palatine glands.*

### d. Cruciform suture

It is formed by the following three sutures.
  i. *Intermaxillary suture.*
  ii. *Interpalatine suture.*
  iii. *Palatomaxillary sutures.*

### e. Incisive fossa

1. It is present anteriorly in the median plane of hard palate.
2. *Incisive foramen* (right and left) pierces its corresponding side.

3. Each incisive foramen is transvered by *nasopalatine nerve* and *greater palatine vessels.*

### f. Greater palatine foramen

1. It is present behind the lateral part of palatomaxillary suture.
2. *Greater palatine vessels and nerve* pass through it.
3. A groove observed between greater palatine foramen and incisive fossa is meant for greater palatine vessels.

### g. Lesser palatine foramina

1. These are 1–3 foramina in the pyramidal process of palatine bone and located just behind the greater palatine foramen on each side.
2. *Lesser palatine nerves and vessels* pass through these foramina.

### h. Palatine crest

1. It is a curved ridge observed in the hard palate near its posterior border.

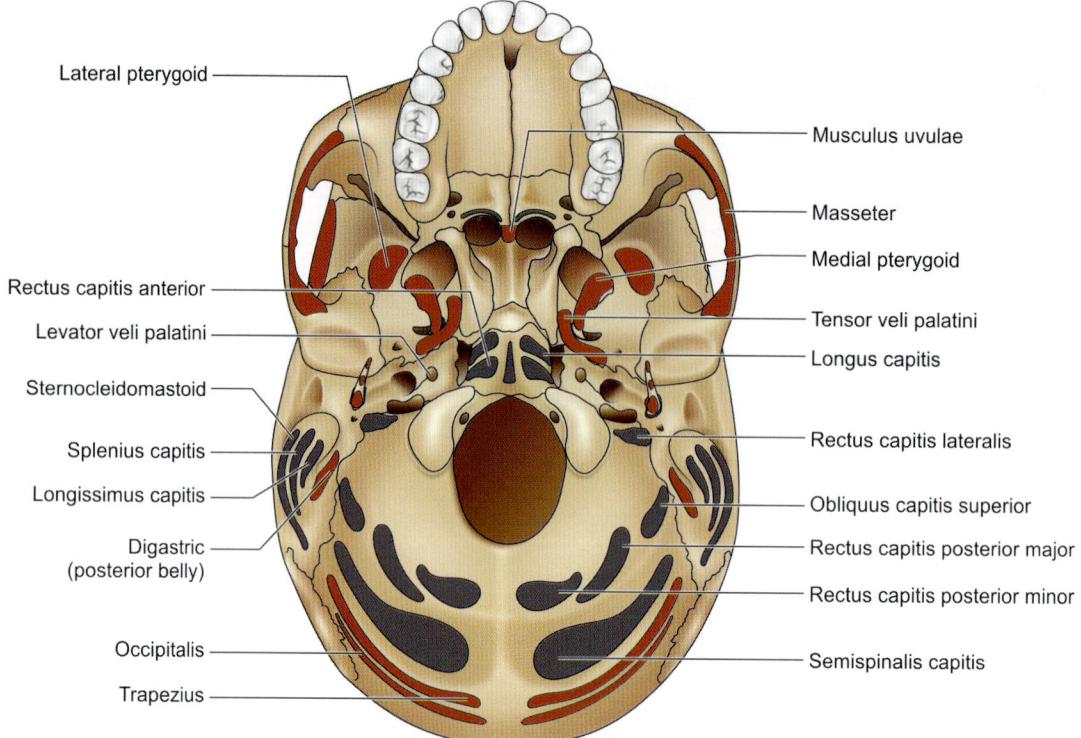

Lateral pterygoid

Musculus uvulae

Masseter

Medial pterygoid

Rectus capitis anterior

Levator veli palatini

Tensor veli palatini

Longus capitis

Sternocleidomastoid

Splenius capitis

Rectus capitis lateralis

Longissimus capitis

Obliquus capitis superior

Digastric (posterior belly)

Rectus capitis posterior major

Rectus capitis posterior minor

Occipitalis

Semispinalis capitis

Trapezius

**Fig. 3.13:** The skull: Norma basalis showing muscular attachments

2. *Palatine aponeurosis* is attached to the palatine crest, posterior border of hard palate and the area between the two.

### i. Premaxilla

1. It is a triangular piece of maxilla holding four incisor teeth.
2. It is a separate bone in most vertebrates.

### B. Middle part of norma basalis

For the sake of convenience, it is divided into a median area and two lateral areas (right and left).

### a. Median area

i. *Posterior nasal apertures*

These are also known as *choanae*.

ii. *Posterior border of vomer*

It separates two choanae.

iii. *Alae of vomer*

1. These are two bony plates formed by the splitting of vomer superiorly.
2. It articulates with the rostrum of sphenoid.

iv. *Vomerovaginal canal*

1. It is formed between the lateral border of each ala of vomer and the vaginal process of the medial pterygoid plate.
2. It transmits *branches of pharyngeal nerve and vessels*.

v. *Palatovaginal canal*

1. It is a canal between *vaginal process of medial pterygoid plate* and *sphenoidal process of the palatine bone*.
2. This canal leads anteriorly into posterior wall of pterygopalatine fossa.
3. It transmits *pharyngeal branches of pterygopalatine ganglion* and *pharyngeal branches of 3rd part of maxillary artery*.

**Note:** *Students are invariably confused as to which is the palatovaginal canal and which one is vomerovaginal canal. To differentiate keep in mind that vaginal process of medial pterygoid plate is common to both but as the palatine bone is anterior to medial pterygoid plate the palatovaginal canal is relatively anterior to vomerovaginal canal.*

 vi. *Broad bar of bone behind the alae*
   1. It is formed by the continuation of inferior surface of body of sphenoid and that of basilar part of occipital bone.
   2. It extends up to *foramen magnum.*
   3. *Pharyngeal tubercle* is a median elevation just in front of foramen magnum. It is better felt than seen.
   4. Pharyngeal tubercle gives attachments to:
      • *Highest fibres of superior constrictor.*
      • *Pharyngeal raphe.*
   5. *Longus capitis* is inserted on the basilar part of occipital bone just lateral to pharyngeal tubercle.
   6. *Rectus capitis anterior* is inserted on each side just in front of occipital condyle.

b. *Lateral area*
  i. *Pterygoid processes*
   1. Pterygoid processes are located just behind the posterior ends of alveolar arch.
   2. Each pterygoid process descends vertically downwards from the junction of body and greater wing of sphenoid.
   3. Pterygoid process consists of a lateral and a medial plate.
   4. Ptergoid plates unite anteriorly in the upper part to enclose a fossa called *pterygoid fossa.*
   5. The lower ununited portions form *pterygoid fissure* which is filled by the pyramidal process of palatine bone.

 6. Anterior surface of pterygoid process forms posterior boundary of *pterygopalatine fossa.*
 7. Lateral surface of lateral pterygoid plate forms medial wall of *infratemporal fossa* and gives origin to lower head of *lateral pterygoid muscle.*
 8. Medial surface of lateral pterygoid plate forms lateral wall of *pterygoid fossa* and gives origin to *deep head of medial pterygoid muscle.*
 9. Lateral surface of medial pterygoid plate forms medial wall of pterygoid fossa and is related to *tensor palati* muscle.
 10. Medial surface of the medial pterygoid plate forms the lateral wall of corresponding posterior nasal aperture.
 11. Posterior border of the medial pterygoid plate shows following features:
    • At its upper end, it splits to enclose *scaphoid fossa* which gives origin to *tensor palati* muscle.
    • Its upper end shows a small projection called *pterygoid tubercle* which lies immediately below the posterior end of *pterygoid canal.*
    • *Pharyngobasilar fascia* is attached to its whole extent while *superior constrictor* arises from its lower part only.
    • A hook like process at its lower end is called *pterygoid hamulus.* Tendon of *tensor palati* winds round this process. *Superior constrictor* and *pterygomandibular raphe* are also attached to it.
    • An angular process projecting from the middle of this margin is called *processus tubarius.* Posterior border above this process is called *notch of auditory tube.* This process and notch support the medial end of *auditory tube.*

ii. *Infratemporal surface of greater wing of sphenoid*
 1. It is pentagonal in shape.
 2. It forms roof of *infratemporal fossa*.
 3. It gives origin to the *upper head of lateral pterygoid muscle*.
 4. It is crossed by *deep temporal* and *masseteric nerves*.
 5. *Spine of sphenoid* is a projection from posteriormost part of infratemporal surface.
 6. *Infratemporal crest* is the lateral limit of infratemporal surface.
 7. From scaphoid fossa to spine of sphenoid, four foramina can be noticed, i.e. *foramen of Vesalius, foramen ovale, canaliculus innominatus* and *foramen spinosum*.

iii. *Foramen ovale*
 1. It is an oval foramen.
 2. It transmits the *mandibular nerve, accessory meningeal artery, lesser petrosal nerve and emissary vein.*

**Note:** *For remembering the structures passing through foramen ovale remember MALE, in which M—Mandibular nerve, A—Accessory meningeal artery, L—Lesser petrosal nerve and E—Emissary vein.*

iv. *Foramen spinosum*
 1. It is situated near the spine of sphenoid, posterolateral to foramen ovale.
 2. It transmits *middle meningeal artery, nervus spinosus* (meningeal branch of mandibular nerve) and *parietal trunk of middle meningeal vein*.

v. *Foramen of Vesalius (sphenoidal emissary foramen)*
 1. It is an infrequently seen foramen between scaphoid fossa and foramen ovale.
 2. It transmits an emissary vein connecting cavernous sinus with pterygoid venous plexus.

vi. *Canaliculus innominatus (foramen innominatum)*
 1. This is also an infrequently seen foramen between foramen ovale and foramen spinosum.
 2. It transmits *lesser petrosal nerve.*

vii. *Spine of sphenoid*
 1. It is related laterally to *auriculotemporal nerve* and medially to *chorda tympani nerve* and *Eustachian tube.*
 2. *Sphenomandibular ligament* is attached to its tip.
 3. Most posterior fibres of *tensor palatini* originate from its anterior surface.

viii. *Sulcus tubae*
 1. It is a groove between posteromedial margin of infratemporal surface of greater wing of sphenoid and inferor surcace the petrous part of temporal bone.
 2. *Cartilaginous part of Eustachian tube* (also called auditory tube or pharyngotympanic tube) occupies this sulcus.

ix. *Inferior surface of petrous part of temporal bone*
 1. It is located just behind the infratemporal surface of greater wing of sphenoid.
 2. Its anteromedial serrated end marks the apex of petrous part.
 3. The quadrilateral area near the apex provides attachment to *levator palati muscle.*
 4. Lower opening of *carotid canal* is located just behind the quadrilateral area. It *transmits internal carotid artery with its sympathetic and venous plexuses.*
 5. Carotid canal runs forwards and medially in petrous part and perforates its apex as upper opening of carotid canal.

x. *Foramen lacerum*
 1. It is located between sphenoid and apex of petrous temporal.

2. It is named *'lacerum'* because of irregular margins.

3. *Carotid canal* and *pterygoid canal* open into it.

4. Only two structures pass through it, i.e. *meningeal branch of ascending pharyngeal artery* and *emissary vein*.

5. *Internal carotid artery* traverses its upper part *with its sympathetic and venous plexuses*.

6. *Nerve of pterygoid canal (Vidian nerve)* is formed in its upper part by the union of *greater superficial petrosal and deep petrosal nerves*.

xi. *Tympanic part of temporal bone*

1. It is a triangular bone which occupies the angle between the petrous and squamous parts of temporal bone.

2. Its anterior surface is related to *parotid gland*.

xii. *Squamous part of temporal bone*

Only a small part of squamous part of temporal bone is seen in norma basalis and shows following features from posterior to anterior:

1. Anterior (articular) part of *mandibular fossa*.

2. *Articular tubercle*.

3. Part of the roof of infratemporal fossa.

xiii. *Squamotympanic fissure*

1. It marks the junction of squamous and tympanic parts of temporal bone.

2. Downward edge of tegmen tympani (a part of petrous part of temporal bone) divides the squamotympanic fissure into *petrotympanic* (posterior) and *pterosquamous* (anterior) *fissures*.

3. *Chorda tympani nerve, anterior tympanic artery* and *anterior ligament of malleus* pass through petrotympanic fissure.

## C. Posterior part of norma basalis

For the sake of convenience this part can be divided into a median area and two lateral areas (right and left).

### a. Median area

It consists of foramen magnum, external occipital crest and external occipital protuberance from anterior to posterior.

i. *Foramen magnum*

1. It is the largest foramen in skull.

2. It is single foramen located in the lowest part of posterior cranial fossa.

3. It is oval in shape.

4. It is the communication between cranial cavity and vertebral canal.

5. *Anterior atlanto-occipital membrane* is attached to its anterior margin.

6. *Posterior atlanto-occipital membrane* is attached to its posterior margin.

7. Lateral margins provide attachments to *alar ligaments*.

8. Following structures pass through its anterior part:
   - *Apical ligament of dens.*
   - *Superior longitudinal band of cruciform ligament.*
   - *Membrana tectoria.*

9. Following structures pass through its posterior part:
   - *Medulla oblongata.*
   - *Meninges.*
   - *Spinal roots of accessory nerves.*
   - *Meningeal branches of upper cervical nerves (C$_{1-3}$).*
   - *Vertebral arteries.*
   - *Sympathetic plexuses around vertebral arteries.*
   - *Anterior and posterior spinal arteries.*

ii. *External occipital crest*

1. It extends from posterior margin of foramen magnum to external occipital protuberance.

2. Upper margin of *ligamentum nuchae* is attached to it.

iii. *External occipital protuberance*

*Trapezius* is attached to it superiorly and *ligamentum nuchae* inferiorly.

b. *Lateral area*

i. *Occipital condyles*

1. These are located lateral to anterior half of foramen magnum.

2. Each is oval and convex to articulate with concave superior articular process of atlas.

ii. *Condylar fossa*

1. It is present just behind the occipital condyle.

2. It may have *condylar canal for emissary vein* from sigmoid sinus.

iii. *Hypoglossal canal*

1. Lateral to anterior part of condyle is the outer opening of hypoglossal canal.

2. It transmits:
   - *Hypoglossal nerve.*
   - *Meningeal branch of ascending pharyngeal artery.*
   - *Emissary vein from basilar venous plexus.*

iv. *Squamous part of occipital bone*

1. *Superior nuchal line* is a well defined ridge which extends laterally from external occipital protuberance on each side. Its medial 1/3rd provides origin to *trapezius* while lateral 1/3rd receives insertions of *sternomastoid* (above) and *splenius capitis* (below).

2. Running laterally on each side from the middle of external occipital crest is another ridge called *inferior nuchal line.*

3. A vertical line on each side along with inferior nuchal line divides the region below the superior nuchal line into four areas, each meant for the attachment of a muscle as follows:
   - Upper medial area for *semispinalis capitis.*
   - Upper lateral area for obliquus capitis superior.
   - Lower medial area for *rectus capitis posterior minor.*
   - Lower lateral area for *rectus capitis posterior major.*

v. *Jugular foramen*

1. It is an interosseous foramen situated between anterior margin of jugular process of occipital bone and posterior margin of petrous part of temporal bone at the petro-occipital suture.

2. It is divided into anterior, middle and posterior parts.

3. *9th, 10th and 11th cranial nerves* pass through its middle part.

4. *Inferior petrosal sinus* and *meningeal branch of ascending pharyngeal artery* pass through its anterior part.

5. *Sigmoid sinus* and *meningeal branch of occipital artery* traverse through its posterior part.

6. At its posterior end the anterior wall (petrous temporal) is hollowed out to form the *jugular fossa* which lodges the superior bulb of internal jugular vein.

7. *Mastoid canaliculus* is a minute canal in the lateral wall of jugular fossa which transmits the *auricular branch of vagus.*

8. *Glossopharyngeal notch* is on the posterior border of petrous temporal bone near the medial end of jugular foramen.

9. *Cochlear canaliculus* is located at the apex of glossopharyngeal notch. The *aqueduct of cochlea* opens into the cochlear canaliculus.

10. *Tympanic canaliculus* is present in the ridge between jugular fossa and lower opening of carotid canal. It transmits the *tympanic branch of glossopharyngeal nerve* to middle ear.

vi. *Inferior surface of jugular process of occipital bone*

1. It is the area just lateral to occipital condyle behind the jugular foramen.

2. It provides attachment to *rectus capitis lateralis*.

vii. *Styloid process*

1. It is a conical projection just below the tympanic part of temporal bone.

2. It is directed downwards, forwards and slightly medially.

3. It provides attachments to 3 muscles and 2 ligaments. Three muscles attached to it are *styloglossus* (anteriorly), *stylohyoid* (posteriorly) and *stylo-pharyngeus* (medially). Two ligaments attached to it are *stylomandibular* (laterally) and *stylohyoid* (on the tip).

4. It is interposed between *parotid gland* (laterally) and *internal jugular vein* (medially).

5. Two structures cross it superficially, i.e. *facial nerve* (near the base) and *external carotid artery* (near the tip).

viii. *Mastoid process*

1. It is a prominent projection from the temporal bone posterolateral to styloid process.

2. The medial aspect of this process shows a deep groove (*digastric notch*)

which provides attachment to *posterior belly of digastric*.

3. Medial to digastric notch, there can be another *groove for occipital artery*.

ix. *Stylomastoid foramen*

1. It is present between styloid and mastoid processes.

2. *Facial nerve* and *stylomastoid artery* pass through this foramen.

## Applied anatomy

1. A forceful hit on the forehead causes linear fracture of both vertex and base (Fig. 3.14).

2. Due to the presence of natural thick bony buttresses at the base of skull, the fracture lines often converge towards the foramen magnum or sella turcica.

3. In case of basal fractures, loceration of structures passing through the basal foramina may complicate the issue.

4. A fracture line passing through the foramen lacerum may tear the internal carotid artery with a resultant *caroticocavernous fistula*.

5. If the fissure lines involve grooves having meningeal vessels and dural sinuses, then *epidural haematoma* might result.

6. Fractures of skull base are often zig-zag in appearance because the fracture lines avoid

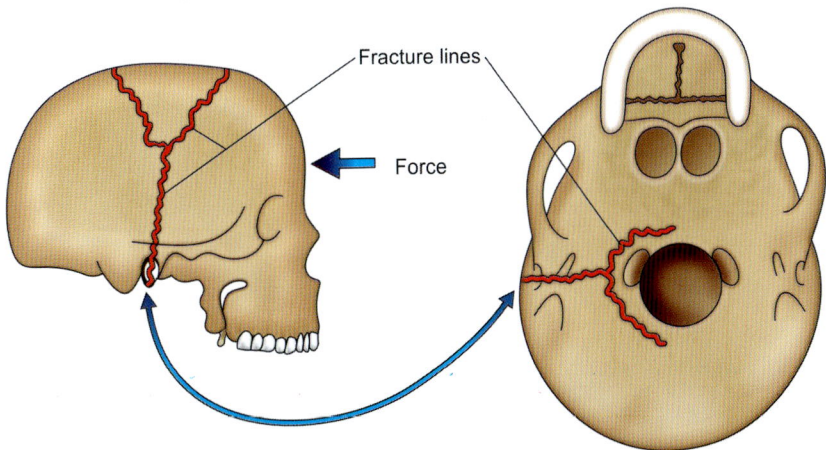

**Fig. 3.14:** Fracture of skull base due to hit on forehead

the thickenings and pass through the lines of least resistance.

7. Tumours of the base of skull

   A. *Transitional cell carcinoma* arising from mucous membrane of paranasal sinuses or fossa of Rosenmuller of nasopharynx usually erodes the skull base.

   B. Some of the very rare tumours which may arise from the base of skull or adjacent tissue, are as follows:

      i. *Osteomas.*

      ii. *Chondromas.*

      iii. *Giant cell tumours of bone.*

   C. Many malignant tumours metastasize to the base of skull bones from distant organs, e.g. prostate, lung and breast.

8. Bony palate may be fractured in uncommon central split of palate. It is actually paramedian in nature because median sutures (intermaxillary and interpalatine) are relatively strong (Fig. 3.15).

9. Clinical signs and symptoms which support the involvement of base of skull, are as follows:

    i. Discharge of CSF through external acoustic meatus (*C.S.F. otorrhoea*)

    ii. Tear of tympanic membrane.

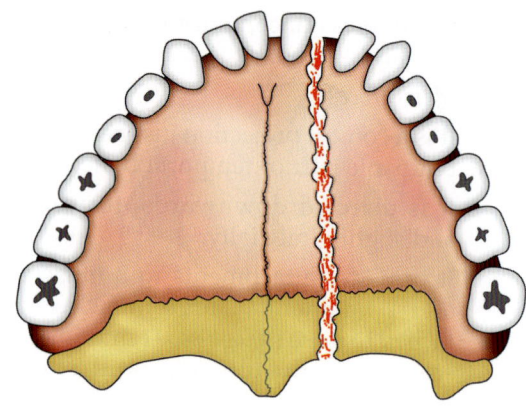

**Fig. 3.15:** Central split of palate

    iii. Collection of blood in the middle ear.

    iv. *Facial paralysis* due to damage of 7th cranial nerve.

    v. Loss of hearing, vertigo and nystagmus due to involvement of 8th cranial nerve. Aforementioned signs are indicative of fracture of petrous part of temporal bone.

    vi. Discolouration and oedema of tissue over mastoid process is indication of sigmoid sinus damage.

10. Cranial nerve damage is due to involvement of foramina in the skull base by the fracture lines.

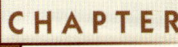

# Orbital Cavity

## DEFINITION

Orbits are two bony sockets which lodge the eyeballs and the associated structures.

## SHAPE AND PARTS (Fig. 4.1)

Each orbit is pyramidal in shape having an anterior base (orbital opening), posterior apex and four walls (medial, lateral, roof and floor).

## BONY CONTRIBUTIONS (Fig. 4.2)

### A. Orbital opening (base)

It consists of four margins (supraorbital, infraorbital, lateral and medial).

### a. Supraorbital margin

1. It is formed by the frontal bone.
2. *Supraorbital notch (or foramen)* is situated at the junction of its medial 1/3rd (rounded) and lateral 2/3rd (sharp) parts.
3. Supraorbital notch transmits:
   i. *Supraorbital nerve.*
   ii. *Supraorbital artery.*
   iii. *Communicating vein between angular and superior ophthalmic veins.*

### b. Infraorbital margin

It is formed by maxilla medially and zygomatic bone laterally.

### c. Lateral orbital margin

It is formed by the frontal process of zygomatic bone below and the zygomatic process of frontal bone above.

### d. Medial orbital margin

It is formed by the frontal bone above and the lacrimal crest of frontal process of maxilla below.

### B. Apex

1. It forms the posterior end of orbit.
2. It is contributed by sphenoid.
3. Usually the medial end of superior orbital fissure is said to mark the apex.

### C. Medial wall

It is formed by the following bones from anterior to posterior:

a. Posterior part of the frontal process of *maxilla.*
b. *Lacrimal bone.*
c. The orbital plate of *ethmoid.*
d. Body of *sphenoid.*

### D. Lateral wall

It is contributed by:

a. *Greater wing of sphenoid bone* posteriorly.
b. *Orbital surface of zygomatic bone* and *medial aspect of its frontal process* anteriorly.

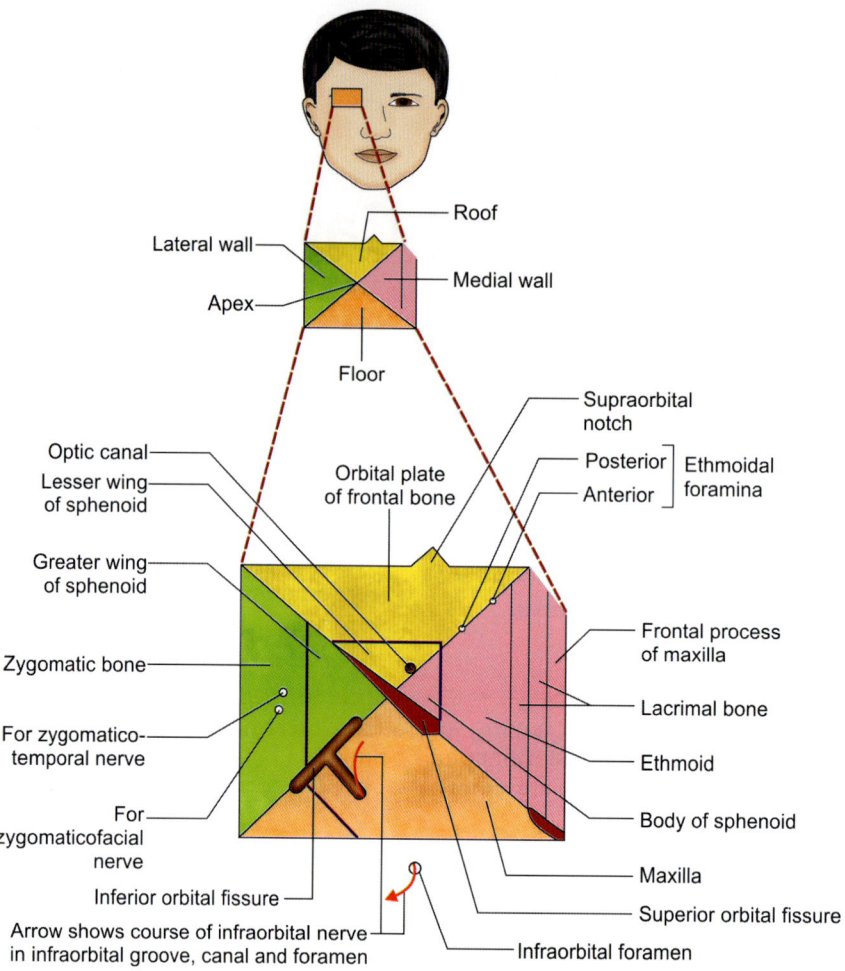

**Fig. 4.1:** Right orbit: Anterior view

## E. Roof

It is formed by:

a. *Orbital plate of frontal bone* anteriorly.

b. *Lesser wing of sphenoid* posteriorly.

## F. Floor

It is formed by:

a. *Orbital surface of maxilla* medially. It is the major contribution.

b. *Orbital surface of zygomatic bone*.

c. *Orbital process of palatine bone*. It is an insignificant contribution near the posterior end at the junction of medial wall and floor.

## COMMUNICATIONS (Fig. 4.3)

The orbit communicates through several passages with adjacent regions as shown below.

| Passages | Adjacent regions |
| --- | --- |
| 1. Orbital opening | Face |
| 2. Infraorbital canal | Face |
| 3. Optic canal | Middle cranial fossa |
| 4. Superior orbital fissure | Middle cranial fossa |
| 5. Inferior orbital fissure | |
|   a. Medially | Pterygopalatine fossa |
|   b. Laterally | Infratemporal fossa |

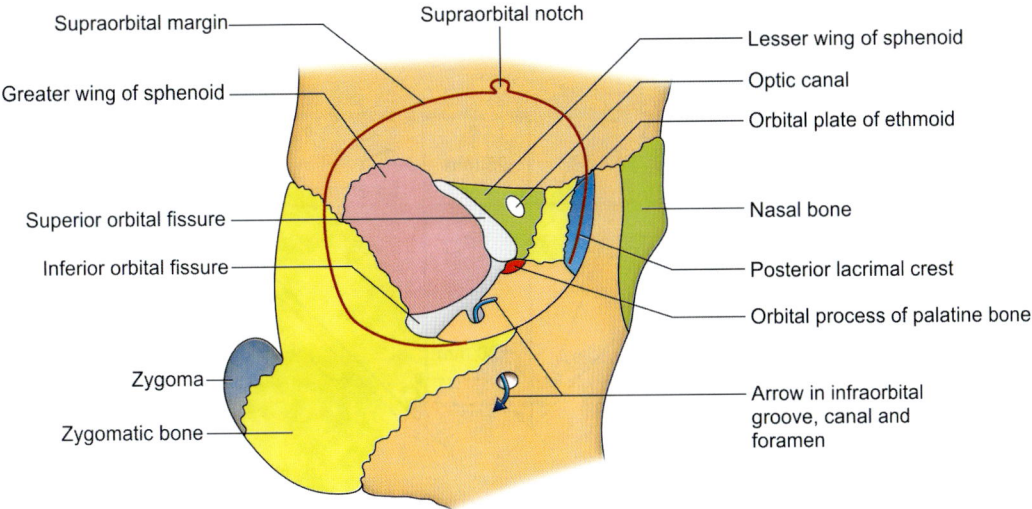

**Fig. 4.2:** Right orbit: Anterior view

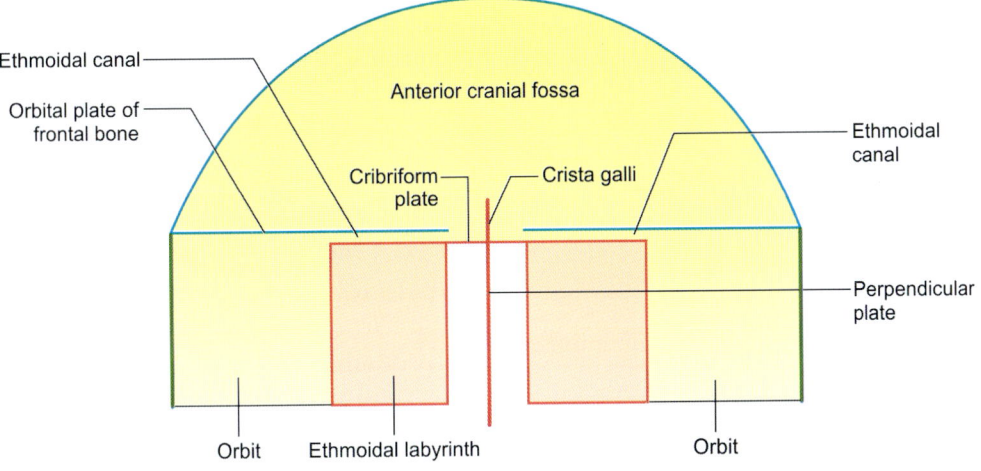

**Fig. 4.3:** Diagramatic representation of ethmoidal canal in coronal sectional view

| 6. Zygomatico-orbital foramina | Face and temporal fossa |
|---|---|
| 7. Anterior and posterior ethmoidal canals | Anterior cranial fossa |
| 8. Nasolacrimal canal | Nasal cavity |

## MEASUREMENTS (Fig. 4.4)

1. Length of medial wall—50 mm.
2. Length of lateral wall—50 mm.
3. Width of orbital opening, i.e. distance between medial and lateral orbital margins—40 mm.
4. Distance between two lateral orbital margins—100 mm.
5. Distance between two medial orbital margins—25 mm.
6. Angle between two lateral walls—90°.
7. Angle between lateral and medial walls of each orbit—45°.

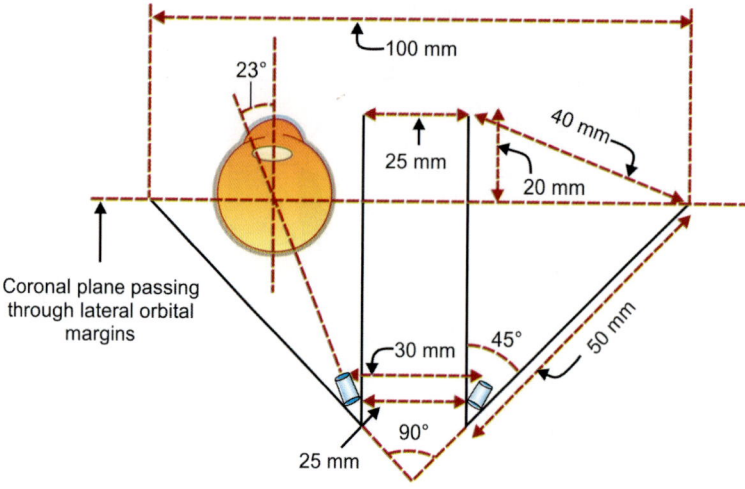

**Fig. 4.4:** Horizontal sectional view of orbits showing measurements

8. Angle between long axis of orbit and anteroposterior axis of eyeball—23°.
9. Distance between medial orbital margin and coronal plane passing through lateral orbital margins—20 mm.
10. Measurements of optic canal:
    i. Length—3–9 mm.
    ii. Diameter—5 mm.
    iii. Distance between orbital openings of optic canals—30 mm.
    iv. Distance between cranial openings of optic canals—25 mm.

## FEATURES

1. Anterolateral part of roof is slightly hollowed out to form *fossa for lacrimal gland*.
2. The anteromedial part of roof near the orbital opening is marked by the *trochlear fovea* or *spine* for the attachment of fibrocartilaginous pulley meant for the tendon of superior oblique muscle.
3. *Optic canal* is present at the posterior end of junction of roof and medial wall. *Optic nerve* and *ophthalmic artery* pass through optic canal.

4. The posterior part of the junction of lateral wall and floor is marked by **inferior orbital fissure**. It transmits the following structures:
   i. *Maxillary nerve.*
   ii. *Infraorbital vessels.*
   iii. *Zygomatic nerve.*
   iv. *A branch from inferior ophthalmic vein.*
   v. *Some twigs (orbital branches) from pterygopalatine ganglion.*
   **Boundaries** of inferior orbital fissure are as follows:
   a. Superiorly—*Greater wing of sphenoid.*
   b. Inferiorly—*Body of maxilla* and *orbital process of palatine bone*
   c. Laterally—*Zygomatic bone.*
5. Maxillary part of the floor is marked by a groove (*infraorbital groove*) in the posterior part. This groove is directed forwards and continues with the *infraorbital canal* in the anterior part of floor and ultimately opens on the face as *infraorbital foramen*. Infraorbital groove, canal and foramen are meant for the passage of infraorbital nerve and vessels.

6. In the anterior part of medial wall, the posterior part of frontal process of maxilla (behind the anterior lacrimal crest) and anterior part of lacrimal bone (anterior to posterior lacrimal crest) form a vertical fossa called *lacrimal fossa*. This fossa continues down with the beginning of *nasolacrimal canal*. The fossa and canal are meant for *lacrimal sac* and *nasolacrimal duct* respectively.

7. *Anterior lacrimal crest* provides attachments to:
   i. *Lacrimal fascia.*
   ii. *Medial palpebral ligament.*
   iii. *Orbicularis oculi.*

8. *Posterior lacrimal crest* gives attachments to:
   i. *Lacrimal fascia.*
   ii. *Lacrimal part of orbicularis occuli.*

9. The junction of orbital plate of frontal bone (roof) and orbital plate of ethmoid (medial wall) shows two openings which lead into *anterior and posterior ethmoidal canals*. These transmit corresponding *ethmoidal nerves and vessels.*

10. Orbital surface of zygomatic bone in the lateral wall possesses *zygomatico-orbital foramina* meant for the passage of *zygomaticotemporal* and *zygomaticofacial nerves* and *zygomatic branches of lacrimal artery.*

11. **Superior orbital fissure**
   A. *Location*
      It is located at the junction of roof and lateral wall of orbit.
   B. *Shape*
      It is triangular in shape with base medially and apex laterally.
   C. *Communication*
      It connects orbit with middle cranial fossa.
   D. *Boundaries*
      i. Medial: *Body of sphenoid bone.*
      ii. Apex: *Frontal bone.*
      iii. Superior: *Lesser wing of sphenoid.*
      iv. Inferior: *Greater wing of sphenoid.*
   E. *Common annular tendon*
      The lower margin of fissure presents a bony projection for the attachment of common tendinous ring (common annular tendon) for the attachment of recti of eyeball.
   F. *Structures passing through*
      Common annular tendon divides the fissure into three compartments for the passage of number of structures as shown below.
      a. Lateral part
         i. *Lacrimal nerve.*
         ii. *Frontal nerve.*
         iii. *Trochlear nerve.*
         iv. *Superior ophthalmic vein.*
         v. *Meningeal branch of lacrimal artery.*
         vi. *Orbital branch of middle meningeal artery.*
      b. Part within tendinous ring
         i. *Upper and lower divisions of the oculomotor nerve.*
         ii. *Nasociliary nerve.*
         iii. *Abducent nerve.*
      c. Part below the tendinous ring
         i. *Inferior ophthalmic vein*
         ii. *Sympathetic twigs.*

12. The lateral wall of orbit near the lateral orbital margin presents an ill defined *Whitnall's tubercle*. It is located on the orbital surface of frontal process of zygomatic bone about 1 cm below the frontozygomatic suture. Following structures are attached to this tubercle:
   i. *Lateral palapebral ligament.*
   ii. *Lateral check ligament.*
   iii. *Suspensory ligament of eyeball.*
   iv. *Aponeurosis of levator palpebrae superioris.*

## APPLIED ANATOMY

1. *Maxillectomy* should be performed below the attachements of check ligaments to avoid the sagging of eyeball (Fig. 4.5).

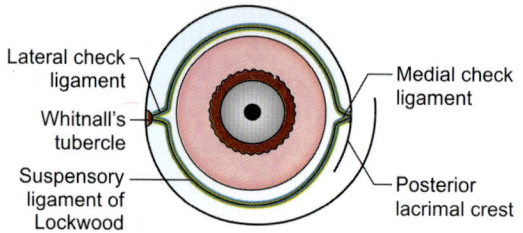

**Fig. 4.5:** Check ligaments located in the right orbit

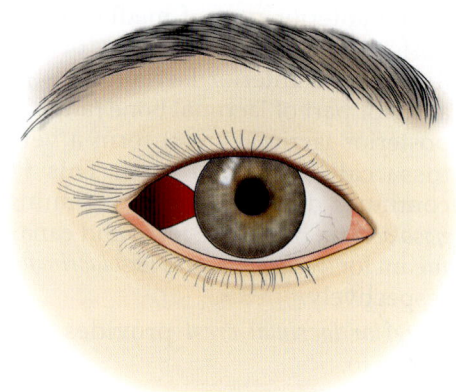

**Fig. 4.6:** Haemorrhage in orbit

2. Normal amount of orbital fat stabilizes the eyeball from behind. An increase in the orbital fat as observed in *hyperthyroidism*, will push the eyeball forwards leading to *exophthalmos* (bulging of eye).

3. The floor and medial wall of the orbit are relatively thin therefore *tumours* arising from ethmoidal and maxillary sinuses may push into the orbital cavity and displace the eyeball.

4. In *Graves' disease* there is hypertrophy of extraocular muscles which is responsible for increased intraorbital pressure and exophthalmos.

5. Eyeball occupies the anterior half of orbit and it is joined by the optic nerve from behind. Optic nerve runs a tortuous course to allow the movements of eyeball without being damaged. Inflammation of optic nerve is called *retrobulbar neuritis.*

6. There may be isolated fracture of single orbital margin or wall or there can be involvement of multiple margins or walls in different combinations.

7. Fracture of the orbital plate of frontal bone causes *haemorrhage* into the orbit. The haemorrhage acquires a triangular shape under the conjunctiva whose apex is towards the corneoscleral junction and base towards the orbital margin (Fig. 4.6).

8. A severe impact on the nasal bridge may involve the medial wall of orbit. Involvement of lacrimal bone will damage the lacrimal passage.

9. A fracture of sphenoid may lacerate the optic nerve in the optic canal resulting into *blindness.*

10. Frontozygomatic suture located in the leteral orbital margin forms an important landmark in the treatment of *maxillofacial injuries.*

11. Fracture of the frontal process of the zygomatic bone may occur in conjunction with a *comminuted fracture* of the orbital rim and frontal bone.

12. Orbit is an anatomical region which is of great clinical and surgical interest due to many disciplines in its surrounding relations.

13. Floor of the orbit is very thin and further weakened by the presence of infraorbital groove. A fracture which is common in this part, invariably involves infraorbital nerve and vessels.

14. *Le Fort (II and III) fractures* of mid-facial skeleton involve the walls of orbit. Fracture line in case of Le Fort II fracture crosses the lower part of frontal process of maxilla and lacrimal bone. In Le Fort III fracture both medial and lateral walls are involved near the roof (Fig. 4.7).

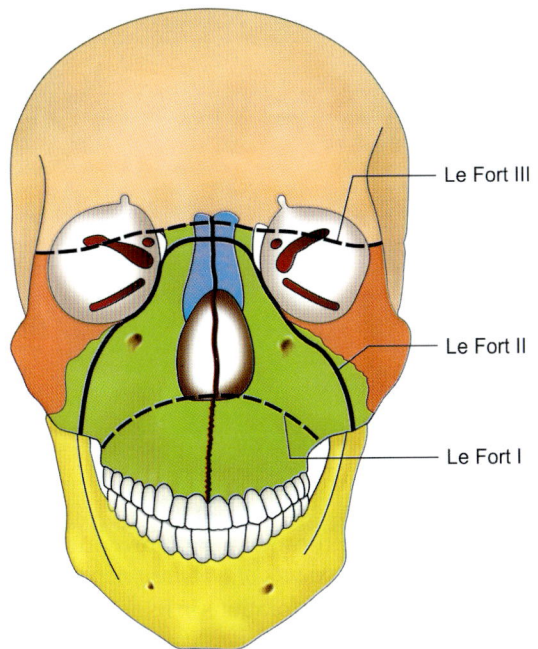

Le Fort III

Le Fort II

Le Fort I

**Fig. 4.7:** Le Fort fractures

15. For *optic nerve decompression* in the optic canal, posterior lacrimal crest, ethmoid and sphenoid are infractured to reach the medial wall of optic canal.

16. Lacrimal bone is very fragile therefore an extra precaution should be taken to avoid trauma in cases of surgery of the lacrimal system.

17. A *penetrating object* will enter the orbit through orbital opening and damage the adjacent regions depending upon its directions, for examples:
    a. Directed upwards and medially: It will enter the frontal sinus in the anterior part and anterior cranial fossa more posteriorly.
    b. Directed towards the floor: It will enter the maxillary sinus.
    c. Directed backwards: It will enter the middle cranial fossa through superior orbital fissure and damage temporal lobe.

18. *Ethmoidal malignancy* may erode the optic canal and compress the optic nerve.

19. *Tumours in the adjacent regions* may enter the orbit through large communications. From middle cranial fossa, it passes through superior orbital fissure while from temporal fossa it traverses the inferior orbital fissure.

20. An *orbital tumour* will push the eyeball forwards producing *exophthalmos*.

21. Since lateral orbital margin is lying relatively more posteriorly than medial orbital margin, a lateral approach is preferred for the operations on eyeball.

# 5

# Nasal Cavity

Nasal cavity is the beginning of respiratory system. It is divided into right and left halves by a midline partition called *nasal septum*. To study the cavity, a sagittal section of skull is considered in which one and half of the skull shows *lateral wall of nasal cavity* and the second half shows *nasal septum*.

## FEATURES

Each half of the nasal cavity consists of a roof, floor, medial wall and lateral wall.

### I. Roof

It has anterior and posterior slopings and middle horizontal part.

#### A. Anterior sloping

It is formed by the *nasal bone* and *nasal spine* of the frontal bone.

#### B. Posterior sloping

1. It is formed by the following bones from anterior to posterior:
   i. Anterior surface of *body of sphenoid*.
   ii. *Ala of vomer*.
   iii. *Sphenoidal process of palatine bone*.
2. It possesses *opening of sphenoidal sinus*.

#### C. Middle horizontal part

1. It is formed by the *cribriform plate* of *ethmoid bone*.

2. Number of foramina in it provide passages for *filaments of olfactory nerve*.
3. One of these perforations in its anterior part transmits *anterior ethmoidal nerve and vessels*.

### II. Floor

1. It is formed by the superior surface of bony palate, i.e. *palatine process of maxilla* and *horizontal plate of palatine bone*.
2. Anteriorly near the septum a small *infundibular opening* leads into *incisive canal*.
3. *Nasopalatine nerve* and *greater palatine* vessels traverse the incisive canal.

### III. Medial wall (Fig. 5.1)

1. It is formed by bony septum in a dried skull.
2. Posteroinferior part of the bony septum is contributed by *vomer*.
3. Its anterosuperior part is formed by *perpendicular plate of ethmoid*.
4. *Nasal crest* (below), *sphenoidal crest* and *rostrum* (above and behind) provide minor contributions to bony septum.
5. A groove on each side of vomer descends downwards and forwards towards incisive canal. It lodges nasopalatine nerve.

### IV. Lateral wall (Fig. 5.2)

1. This is very irregular.
2. This is marked by three bracket like projections which run anteroposteriorly

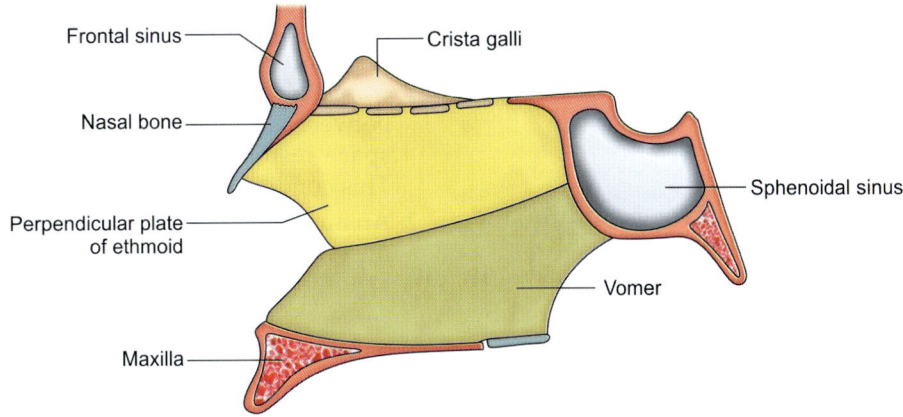

**Fig. 5.1:** Left surface of bony nasal septum

and lie one above the other. These projections are named from above downwards, *superior, middle and inferior conchae.*

3. Each concha forms medial wall and roof of corresponding meatus. Therefore, there are three *meatus, superior, middle and inferior.*

4. The part of the lateral wall above the superior concha is called *sphenoethmoidal recess.*

5. Main bony contributions in the lateral wall are as follows:
   i. Below and in front—*Nasal surface of maxilla.*
   ii. Behind—*Perpendicular plate of palatine bone.*
   iii. Above—*Ethmoidal labyrinth* (with superior and middle conchae).
   iv. Below—*Inferior concha* (an independent bone).

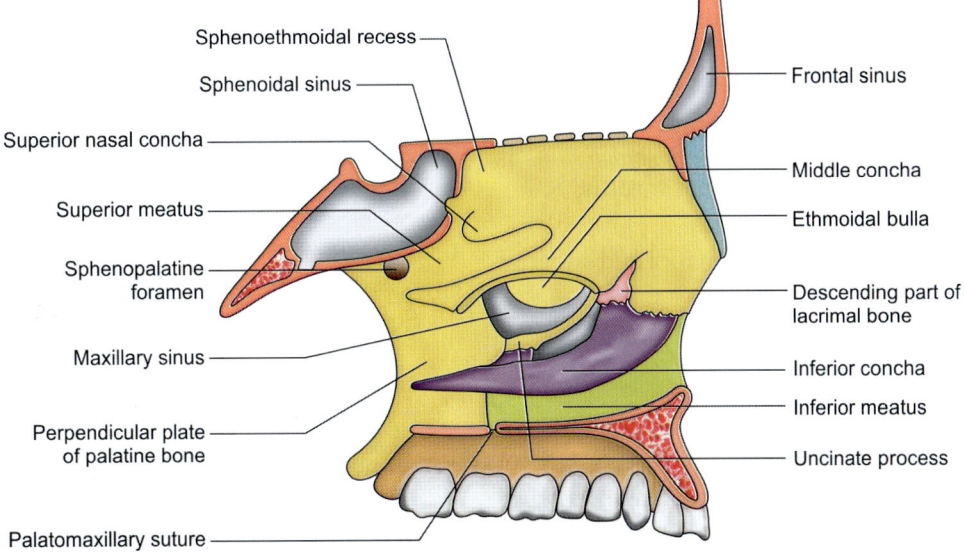

**Fig. 5.2:** Lateral wall of left nasal cavity

6. *Inferior meatus*
   a. It lies below and lateral to inferior concha.
   b. It receives *opening of nasolacrimal duct* in its anterior part.

7. *Middle meatus*
   i. It is situated between middle and inferior conchae.
   ii. A rounded elevation in its upper part is called *ethmoidal bulla* produced by middle ethmoidal air cells.
   iii. On the surface or just above the bulla is the *opening of middle ethmoidal sinus*.
   iv. Behind the bulla is the *opening of maxillary* sinus.
   v. Anteroinferior to bulla is a curved, thin bony projection is called *uncinate process of ethmoid*.
   vi. Uncinate process passes backwards and encloses a curved gap between it and bulla. This gap is called *hiatus semilunaris*.
   vii. Upper end of hiatus semilunaris continues with *ethmoidal infundibulum*.
   viii. Infundibulum of ethmoid receives *opening of anterior ethmoidal sinus* and itself continues up as *frontonasal duct* to reach the frontal sinus.

8. *Superior meatus*
   i. It is situated between superior and middle conchae.
   ii. *Opening of posterior ethmoidal sinus* is located in the superior meatus.

9. *Sphenoethmoidal recess*
   i. It is situated between roof and superior concha.
   ii. It receives the *opening of sphenoidal air sinus*.

10. *Sphenopalatine foramen*
   i. It is located just behind the superior concha.
   ii. It transmits *sphenopalatine artery* and *nasal branches of pterygopalatine ganglion*.

## APPLIED ANATOMY

1. Fracture of base of skull involving anterior cranial fossa might lead to communication between nasal cavity and subarachnoid space resulting CSF leak into the nose. This condition is called *CSF rhinorrhoea*.

2. An impact on the nasal bridge will lead to fracture and displacement of nasal septum.

3. Fracture of cribriform plate will result into *anosmia* (loss of smell sensation) due to damage of olfactory nerve filaments.

4. Fracture of cribriform plate may cause infection to enter the cranial cavity from nasal cavity resulting into *meningitis*.

5. *Le Fort fractures* of mid-facial skeleton always involve the nasal septum (Fig. 5.3).

6. All the bones of nasal cavity are clothed in mucosa, therefore, their fractures open to nasal cavity with potential risk of infection.

7. The bones of nasal cavity receive adequate blood supply from periosteal arteries and, therefore, all the fragments of fractured bone retain a periosteal blood supply.

8. Bony septum is papery thin and does not resist much to forces responsible for fracture.

9. Floor of the nasal cavity may be fractured in uncommon central split of the palate. It is actually paramedian in nature

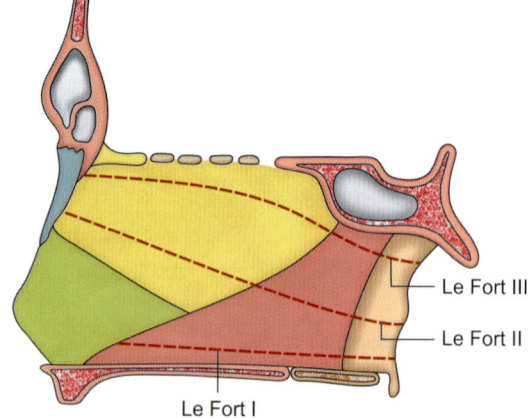

**Fig.5.3:** Fracture lines of Le Fort fractures crossing the nasal septum

because median sutures (intermaxillary and interpalatine) are relatively strong.

10. *Nasal ethmoidostomy* (an artificial opening to drain the ethmoidal air cell) is a common practice in several surgical procedures involving ethmoidal labyrinth.

11. Lacrimal bone is very fragile therefore an extra-precaution should be taken to avoid trauma in cases of surgery of the lacrimal system.

12. In the management of congenital lacrimal defect, *infracture of the inferior concha* is some times needed (Fig. 5.4).

13. In cases of obstruction of lacrimal sac or nasolacrimal duct, *dacryocystorhinostomy* is performed. In this operation an artificial passage is made by breaking lacrimal bone.

14. *Congenital atresia of the choanae* is an uncommon condition in which there is occlusion of the posterior naris by a bony or membranous diaphragm.

15. *Antral puncture* is a common procedure performed by ENT surgeons to wash out infected fluid in maxillary sinus (*antral lavage*). The antrum is punctured through the inferior meatus by a trocar and cannula (Fig. 5.5).

16. *Deviation of nasal septum (DNS)* is a common condition which may be developmental in origin or may arise from trauma.

17. A *perforated septum* may be due to septal surgery or syphilis or tuberculosis.

18. Some times a permanent opening is made in the inferior meatus to encourage the drainage of the pus in the maxillary sinus. This operation is called *intranasal antrostomy*.

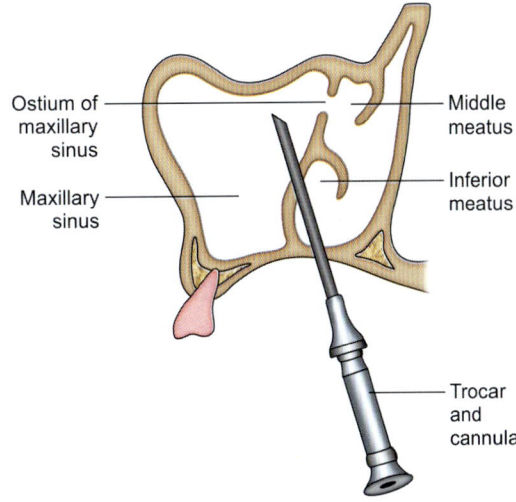

**Fig. 5.5:** Antral puncture

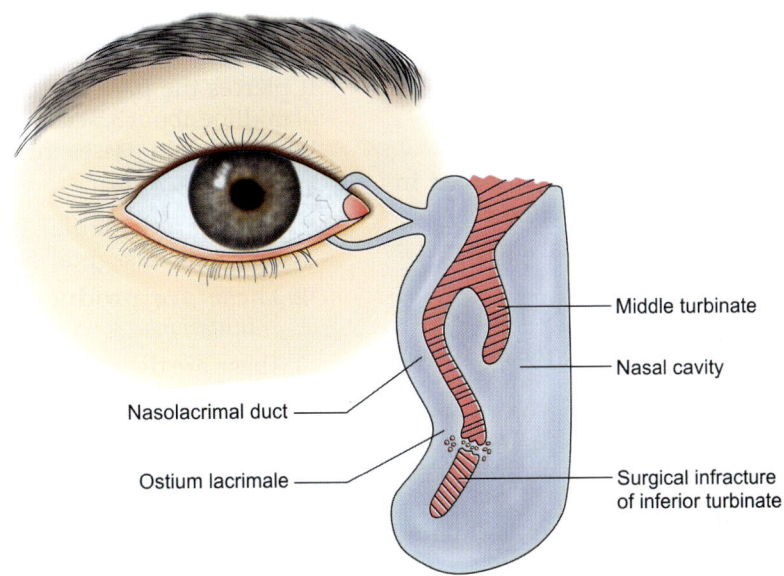

**Fig. 5.4:** Infracture of inferior concha

# 6

# Interior of the Cranial Vault

## DEFINITION

It is the internal surface of the skull cap.

## SHAPE

This is ovoid like norma verticalis.

## BONES

Same bones contribute to this part which were observed in norma verticalis, i.e.

1. Frontal bone, anteriorly.
2. Occipital bone, posteriorly
3. Parietal bones, on each side.

## SUTURES

Sutures correspond with those observed in norma verticalis which are as follows:

1. *Coronal suture*, between frontal and parietal bones.
2. *Sagittal suture*, between two parietal bones.
3. *Lambdoid suture*, between parietal and occipital bones.

## FEATURES (Fig. 6.1)

### A. Frontal crest
1. It is a midline crest seen at its anterior part.
2. *Falx cerebri* is attached to it.

### B. Sagittal sulcus
1. It is an anteroposterior groove in the median plane.
2. It is narrow anteriorly but widens posteriorly.
3. It contains superior *sagittal sinus*.
4. *Falx cerebri* is attached to its margins.

### C. Bregma and lambda
These mark the junctions of sagittal suture with coronal and lambdoid sutures respectively (see norma verticalis).

### D. Parietal foramen
It pierces the parietal bone on each side of midline about 3.5 cm in front of lambda. Emissary vein passes through it.

### E. Granular foveolae
1. These are irregular depressions on each side of sagittal sulcus.
2. These are produced by *arachnoid granulations*.
3. These are deep and more abundant in aged skull.

### F. Grooves for meningeal vessels
1. Grooves for anterior (frontal) twigs of middle meningeal vessels are located just behind the coronal suture.
2. Grooves for parietal twigs of middle meningeal vessels are more posteriorly

44

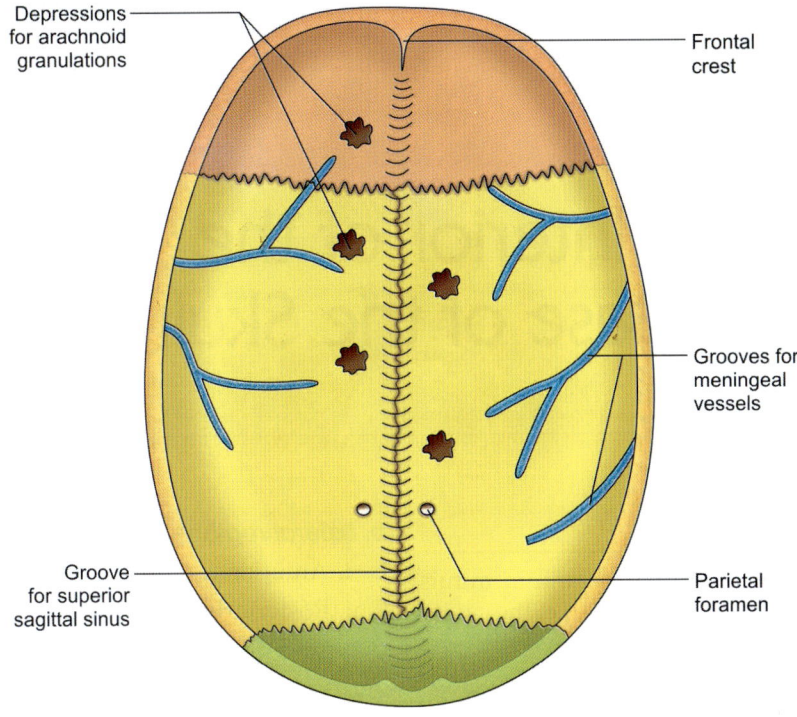

Depressions for arachnoid granulations

Frontal crest

Grooves for meningeal vessels

Groove for superior sagittal sinus

Parietal foramen

**Fig. 6.1:** Skull cap: Internal surface

placed. These run backwards and upwards.

### G. Impressions for cerebral gyri

These are less marked in cranial vault in contrast to the interior of the base of skull where cerebral impressions are well defined.

### APPLIED ANATOMY

For details *see* page 12 of applied anatomy in norma verticalis.

# Interior of the Base of the Skull

## DEFINITION

It is the base of skull (neurocranium minus skull cap) observed from inside, i.e. the cavity side.

## SUBDIVISIONS

Internal surface of the base of the skull is naturally demarcated into three fossae known as the anterior, middle and posterior cranial fossae.

## I. ANTERIOR CRANIAL FOSSA

### A. Boundaries

#### a. Anterior and lateral

*Frontal bone.*

#### b. Posterior

  i. *Posterior border of lesser wing of sphenoid.*
  ii. *Anterior clinoid process.*
  iii. *Anterior margin* of *sulcus chiasmatis.*

### B. Floor

#### a. Median region

  i. Anteriorly: *Cribriform plate of ethmoid.*
  ii. Posteriorly: Anterior part of superior surface of body of sphenoid (*jugum sphenoidale*).

#### b. Lateral region

  i. Anteriorly: *Orbital plates of frontal bone.*
  ii. Posteriorly: *Lesser wings of sphenoid.*

### C. Features and attachments (Figs 7.1 and 7.2)

#### a. Frontal crest

1. It is a median crest in the anterior wall of fossa.
2. It provides attachment to *falx cerebri.*

#### b. Crista galli of cribriform plate

1. It is an upward tooth like projection in the midline of cribriform plate just behind the frontal crest.
2. This projection receives attachment of *anterior end of falx cerebri.*

#### c. Foramen caecum

1. It is situated between crista galli and crest of frontal bone.
2. It is usually blind but some times may transmit an *emissary vein* from nasal cavity to superior sagittal sinus.

#### d. Cribriform plate of ethmoid on each side of crista galli

1. It is a sieve-like (perforated) bony plate.

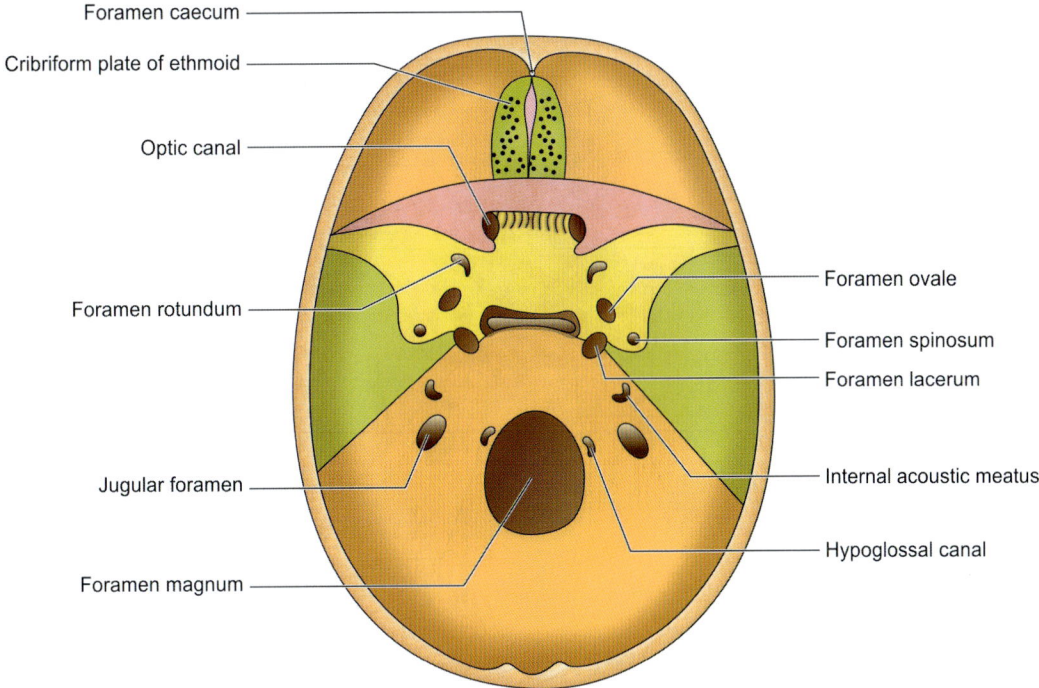

**Fig. 7.1:** Base of skull: Internal surface

2. 15–20 filaments of *olfactory nerve* pass through each perforate plate from olfactory mucosa of nose to olfactory bulb.
3. Groove just lateral to crista galli is related to:
    i. *Olfactory bulb.*
    ii. *Gyrus rectus.*
4. Anterior ethmoidal canal
    i. It opens in the *cribrofrontal suture* behind the crista galli.
    ii. *Anterior ethmoidal nerve and vessels* pass through it.
5. A *slit like aperture* by the side of anterior part of crista galli is meant for a process of dura mater.
6. A foramen just lateral to anterior end of slit.
    Through this passage, *anterior ethmoidal nerve and vessels* enter the nose from anterior cranial fossa.

7. Posterior ethmoidal canal
    i. It is present in the posterolateral corner of cribriform plate.
    ii. It transmits *posterior ethmoidal vessels.*

### e. Jugum sphenoidale

1. It is most anterior part of the superior surface of body of sphenoid.
2. Its anterior margin meets the posterior margin of cribriform plate.
3. Posteriorly it is limited by sulcus chiasmatis.
4. It separates anterior cranial fossa from two sphenoidal sinuses located in the body of sphenoid.

### f. Orbital plates of frontal bone

1. Each of the two orbital plates separates anterior cranial fossa from corresponding orbit just lateral to cribriform plate.

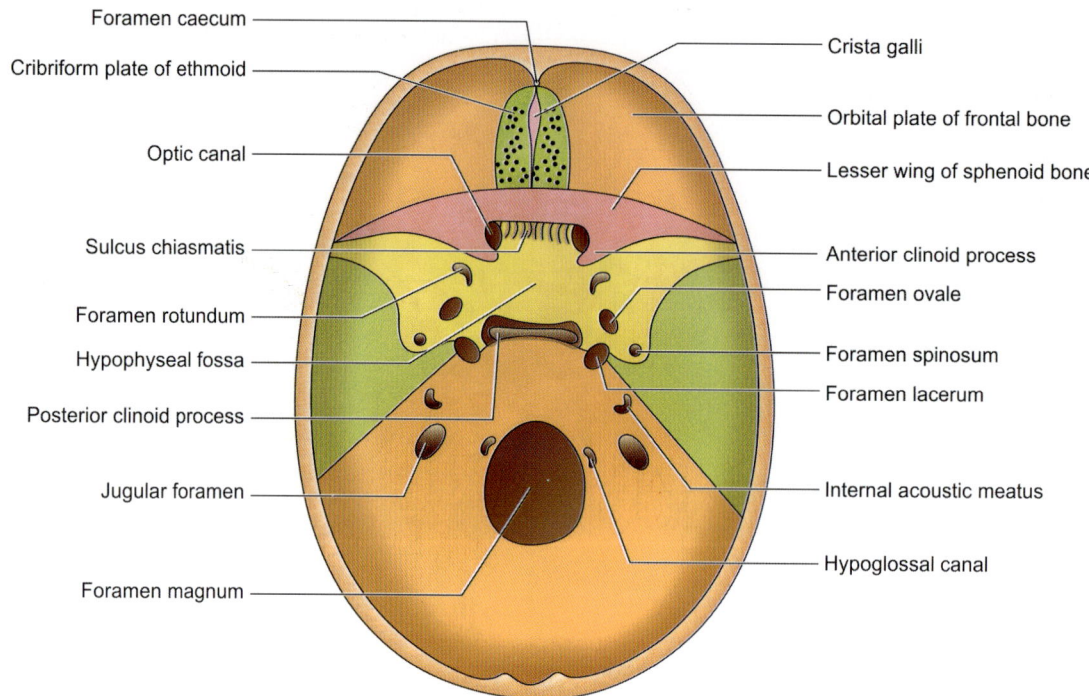

Foramen caecum

Cribriform plate of ethmoid

Optic canal

Sulcus chiasmatis

Foramen rotundum

Hypophyseal fossa

Posterior clinoid process

Jugular foramen

Foramen magnum

Crista galli

Orbital plate of frontal bone

Lesser wing of sphenoid bone

Anterior clinoid process

Foramen ovale

Foramen spinosum

Foramen lacerum

Internal acoustic meatus

Hypoglossal canal

**Fig. 7.2:** Base of skull: Internal surface

2. It shows impressions for cerebral gyri.
3. It supports the orbital surface of frontal lobe of cerebrum.
4. Medially it covers the superior surface of ethmoidal labyrinth (anterior and posterior ethmoidal canals intervening between the two).
5. Posteriorly it meets the anterior margin of lesser wing of sphenoid.

### g. Lesser wings of sphenoid

1. Jugum sphenoidale continues laterally with superior surface of lesser wing.
2. It is broad medially and tapers laterally.
3. Posterior margin of lesser wing is related to:
   i. *Sphenoparietal sinus.*
   ii. *Lateral sulcus* of cerebral hemisphere.
4. Posterior border of lesser wing ends medially into *anterior clinoid process* which receives attachment of free margin of tentorium cerebelli.

## II. MIDDLE CRANIAL FOSSA

### A. Boundaries

#### a. Anterior

i. Posterior border of *lesser wing of sphenoid.*
ii. *Anterior clinoid process.*
iii. Anterior border of *sulcus chiasmatis.*

#### b. Posterior

i. Superior border of *petrous part of temporal bone.*
ii. *Posterior clinoid process.*
iii. *Dorsum sellae.*

#### c. Lateral (on each side)

i. *Greater wing of sphenoid.*
ii. Anteroinferior angle of *parietal bone.*
iii. Squamous part of *temporal bone.*

## B. Floor

### a. Central portion

Body of sphenoid.

### b. Lateral portion (on each side)

i.   *Greater wing of sphenoid.*
ii.  *Squamous part of temporal bone.*
iii. *Anterior surface of petrous temporal.*

## C. Features and attachments

### a. Sulcus chiasmatis

1. It is transversely running groove just behind the jugum sphenoidale.
2. It is named after its relation with the *optic chiasma* which never comes in contact with it but lies posterosuperior to sulcus.
3. Sulcus chiasmatis leads laterally into optic canals.

### b. Optic canal

1. It connects the middle cranial fossa with the orbit.
2. It is bounded by anterior and posterior roots of lesser wing and body of sphenoid.
3. It transmits:
   i.   *Optic nerve.*
   ii.  *Ophthalmic artery.*
   iii. *Meninges.*

### c. Tuberculum sellae

1. It forms an elevation just behind the sulcus chiasmatis.
2. *Middle clinoid processes* are the lateral prominent ends of tuberculum sellae.
3. It receives attachment of anterior margin of *diaphragma sellae.*

### d. Sella turcica

1. It is the depressed area behind the tuberculum sellae.
2. It is shaped like a Turkish saddle and, therefore, named as sella turcica.
3. *Hypophyseal fossa* is the deepest part in it.

It lodges *pituitary gland.*
4. *Sphenoidal air sinus* is present below the floor of the hypophyseal fossa.

### e. Dorsum sellae

1. It is the back of Turkish saddle.
2. It is the square plate of bone behind the sella turcica.
3. Superior angles of dorsum sellae project laterally into *posterior clinoid processes.*
4. *Diaphragma sellae* is attached to the upper margin of dorsum sellae.
5. Anterior end of attached margin of *tentorium cerebelli* is attached to posterior clinoid process.

### f. Carotid sulcus

1. It is observed as a shallow groove on each side of the body of sphenoid.
2. It lodges *cavernous sinus* enclosing cavernous part of *internal carotid artery.*
3. It extends posteriorly up to foramen lacerum where it is deepened.
4. The lateral margin of carotid sulcus at its posterior end, projects backwards into tongue shaped *lingula.*
5. Lingula lies over the *posterior opening of pterygoid canal.*

### g. Superior orbital fissure

1. It is a triangular fissure connecting the lateral portion of middle cranial fossa with orbit.
2. It is bounded above by the *lesser wing*, below by the *greater wing* and medially by the *body of sphenoid.*
3. Common annular tendon (tendinous ring of Zinn) is attached to a small projection seen on the lower border of fissure.
4. Common annular tendon divides the fissure into lateral, middle and medial parts through which following structures traverse:

Through lateral part
   i. *Lacrimal nerve.*

  ii. *Frontal nerve.*

  iii. *Trochlear nerve.*

  iv. *Superior ophthalmic vein.*

  v. *Meningeal branch of lacrimal artery.*

  vi. *Orbital branch of middle meningeal artery.*

Through common annular tendon, i.e. middle part

  i. Upper and lower divisions of *oculomotor nerve.*

  ii. *Nasociliary nerve.*

  iii. *Abducent nerve.*

Through medial part

  i. *Inferior ophthalmic vein.*

  ii. *Sympathetic twigs* form internal carotid sympathetic plexus.

**Note:** *To remember structures passing through superior orbital fissure, remember 'I Slept One Night and Left for Tokyo' in which I—Inferior ophthalmic vein, S—Sympathetic twigs, Superior ophthalmic vein; O—Oculomotor nerve, N—Nasociliary nerve, A—Abducent nerve, L—Lacrimal nerve, F—Frontal nerve, T—Trochlear nerve.*

### h. Foramen rotundum

1. It is present in the greater wing of sphenoid.
2. It is located just below and behind the medial end of superior orbital fissure.
3. It leads forwards into pterygopalatine fossa.
4. It transmits *maxillary nerve.*

**Note:** *Remember, it is not visible in norma basalis.*

### i. Foramen ovale

1. It is located posterolateral to foramen rotundum.
2. It leads inferiorly into infratemporal fossa.
3. It transmits:

  i. *Mandibular nerve.*

  ii. *Accessory meningeal artery.*

  iii. *Lesser petrosal nerve.*

  iv. *Emissary vein.*

**Note:** *Remember ovale: MALE, where M— Mandibular, A—Accessory, L—Lesser and E— Emissary.*

### j. Foramen spinosum

1. It is situated posterolateral to foramen ovale.
2. It leads inferiorly into infratemporal fossa.
3. It transmits:

  i. *Middle meningeal artery.*

  ii. *Nervus spinosus.*

  iii. *Parietal trunk of middle meningeal vein.*

### k. Foramen of Vesalius (sphenoidal emissary foramen)

1. It is inconstant.
2. It is located between foramen rotundum and foramen ovale.
3. It transmits emissary vein connecting the cavernous sinus and pterygoid venous plexus.

### l. Foramen innominatum

1. This is also an inconstant foramen.
2. It is located between foramen ovale and foramen spinosum.
3. It transmits *lesser petrosal nerve.*

### m. Foramen lacerum

1. It is a foramen with irregular margin between sphenoid and apex of petrous temporal.
2. *Carotid* and *pterygoid canals* open into it.
3. Only two structures pass through it, i.e. *meningeal branch of ascending pharyngeal artery* and *emissary vein.*
4. *Internal carotid artery* traverses its upper part *with its sympathetic and venous plexuses.*

5. *Nerve of pterygoid canal* (*Vidian nerve*) is formed in its upper part by the union of *greater superficial petrosal* and *deep petrosal nerves.*

### n. Anterior surface of petrous temporal

1. *Trigeminal impression* is a depression for trigeminal ganglion adjacent to apex.
2. A ridge limits the trigeminal impression posteriorly.
3. *Roof of internal acoustic meatus* is a depressed area behind the ridge.
4. *Arcuate eminence* is a prominent elevation behind the second depression. It is produced by superior semicircular canal. Its posterior sloping lies over lateral and posterior semicircular canals.
5. Area anterolateral to trigeminal impression forms the *roof of anterior part of carotid canal.*
6. Area anterolateral to arcuate eminence forms *roof of vestibule and beginning of facial canal.*
7. Thin plate of bone between squamous temporal and features described above is called *tegmen tympani.* It forms roof of mastoid antrum, middle ear and canal for tensor tympani from posterior to anterior. Tegmen tympani projects downwards to form lateral walls of canal for tensor tympani and bony Eustachian tube and appears in norma basalis in the squamotympanic fissure.
8. A hiatus lateral to arcuate eminence leads into a *groove for greater superficial petrosal nerve* which runs towards foramen laerum on the tegmen tympani.
9. Lateral to aforementioned groove is present another *groove for lesser petrosal nerve* which runs towards foramen ovale.

### o. Superior border of petrous temporal

1. It is gooved by the superior petrosal sinus.
2. Margins of groove provide attachment to tentorium cerebelli.

3. It is crossed by the trigeminal nerve near the apex of petrous temporal.

### p. Lateral part of the fossa shows following additional features

1. Markings for the middle meningeal vessels.
2. Depressions produced by the gyri of temporal lobe of cerebral hemisphere.

## III. POSTERIOR CRANIAL FOSSA

It is largest and the deepest of all cranial fossae. It lodges cerebellum, pons and medulla.

### A. Boundaries

### a. Anterior

   i. *Dorsum sellae.*
   ii. *Posterior clinoid process.*
   iii. *Superior border of petrous temporal.*

### b. Posterior

*Squamous part of occipital bone.*

### c. Lateral

   i. *Mastoid part of temporal bone.*
   ii. Mastoid angle of parietal bone.

### B. Floor

1. *Basisphenoid and basiocciput.*
2. Posterior surface of *petrous temporal.*
3. Mastoid part of *temporal bone.*
4. Posteroinferior angle of the *parietal bone.*
5. Squamous part of *occipital bone.*

### C. Features and attachments

### a. Clivus

1. It is sloping surface in front of foramen magnum.
2. It is formed by the superior surface of basilar part of occipital bone, posterior part of superior surface of body of sphenoid and dorsum sellae.
3. It supports *pons* and *medulla.*

4. It is related to *basilar plexus of veins* and *basilar artery*.

5. Its lower part receives attachments of following structures from above downwards:

   i. *Membrana tectoria.*

   ii. *Superior longitudinal band of cruciform ligament.*

   iii. *Apical ligament of dens.*

### b. Petro-occipital fissure

1. It is the junction between clivus and petrous temporal.

2. It is grooved by the *inferior petrosal sinus.*

### c. Foramen magnum

1. It is largest foramen.

2. It is located in the floor of posterior cranial fossa.

3. Its margins provide attachments to following structures:

   i. *Anterior margin: Anterior atlanto-occipital membrane.*

   ii. *Posterior margin: Posterior atlanto-occipital membrane.*

   iii. *Lateral margins: Alar ligaments.*

4. Structures passing through its anterior part are:

   i. *Apical ligament of dens.*

   ii. *Superior longitudinal band of cruciform ligament.*

   iii. *Membrana tectoria.*

5. Structures passing through its posterior part are:

   i. *Medulla oblongata.*

   ii. *Meninges.*

   iii. *Spinal roots of accessory nerves.*

   iv. *Meningeal branches of upper cervical nerves.*

   v. *Vertebral arteries.*

   vi. *Sympathetic plexuses around the vertebral arteries.*

   vii. *Anterior and posterior spinal arteries.*

### d. Internal occipital protuberance

1. It is situated opposite the external occipital protuberance.

2. It is related to *confluence of dural venous sinuses.*

3. On each side it is grooved by *transverse sinus.*

### e. Internal occipital crest

1. It is a midline crest between internal occipital protuberance and the foramen magnum.

2. *Falx cerebelli* is attached to it.

3. *Cerebellar hemisphere* occupies the deep fossa on each side of the internal occipital crest.

### f. Vermian fossa

1. It is a midline fossa at the lower end of internal occipital crest adjacent to foramen magnum.

2. It is related to *inferior vermis of the cerebellum.*

### g. Transverse sulcus

1. It runs laterally on each side from the internal occipital protuberance.

2. At the mastoid angle of the parietal bone it continues as sigmoid sulcus.

3. It lodges the *transverse sinus.*

4. *Attached margin of tentorium cerebelli* is attached to its lips.

5. Right transverse sulcus is wider than the left one and is continuous posteriorly with superior sagittal sulcus.

### h. Sigmoid sulcus

1. It is downward continuation of transverse sulcus at the mastoid angle of parietal bone.

2. It ends at the lateral end of jugular foramen.

3. It lodges *sigmoid sinus* which enters the jugular foramen to continue with internal jugular vein.

## i. Jugular foramen

1. It is located at the posterior end of *petro-occipital fissure*.

2. It is an interosseous foramen situated between the anterior margin of jugular process of occipital bone and posterior margin of petrous part of temporal bone.

3. It is divided into anterior, middle and posterior parts.

4. *9th, 10th and 11th cranial nerves* pass through its middle part.

5. *Inferior petrosal sinus* and *meningeal branch of ascending pharyngeal artery* traverse its anterior part.

6. Sigmoid sinus and meningeal branch of occipital artery pass through its posterior part.

## j. Jugular tubercle

1. Medial to the lower margin of jugular foramen there is a rounded elevation known as *jugular tubercle*.

2. It is located anterosuperior to the internal opening of hypoglossal canal.

3. It is grooved by the 9th, 10th and 11th cranial nerves.

## k. Hypoglossal canal

1. Its internal opening is located just above the tubercle for alar ligament on the medial aspect of occipital condyle.

2. It transmits:
   i. *Hypoglossal nerve.*
   ii. *Meningeal branch of ascending pharyngeal artery.*
   iii. *Emissary vein from basilar venous plexus.*

## l. Condylar canal

1. It is inconstant.

2. Its internal orifice is located postero-lateral to that of hypoglossal canal.

3. It transmits emissary vein from sigmoid sinus.

## m. Internal acoustic meatus

1. Its *porus* (inlet or medial end) is present in the centre of the posterior surface of petrous temporal.

2. It is about 1 cm in length.

3. It transmits:
   i. *Facial nerve.*
   ii. *Vestibulocochlear nerve.*
   iii. *Labyrinthine vessels.*

4. *Fundus* of internal acoustic meatus is a plate of bone at its lateral end. The plate is divided into upper and lower areas by a transverse ridge (*crista falciformis*). The upper area is further divided into anterior and posterior areas by a vertical crest called *Bill's bar*. Anterior to bar is the *facial canal* for facial nerve. Area behind the bar is called *superior vestibular area* which presents number of small openings for the nerve fibres supplying utricle and superior and lateral semicircular ducts.

Below the transverse crest, anteriorly is the *cochlear area* (which possesses number of foramina called *tractus spiralis foraminosus*) and posteriorly is the *inferior vestibular area*. Fibres of cochlear nerve enter the cochlear area while nerve fibres supplying the saccule enter the inferior vestibular area. Below and behind the inferior vestibular area is *foramen singulare* for the passage of nerve to posterior semicircular duct (Fig. 6.3).

## n. Aqueduct of vestibule

1. A slit behind the porus of internal acoustic meatus leads into aqueduct of vestibule.

2. Aqueduct of vestibule contains *saccus and ductus endolymphaticus along with the small artery and vein.*

## o. Subarcuate fossa

1. It is an irregular depression located above and between the openings of internal acoustic meatus and aqueduct of vestibule.

2. It lodges a process of dura mater.

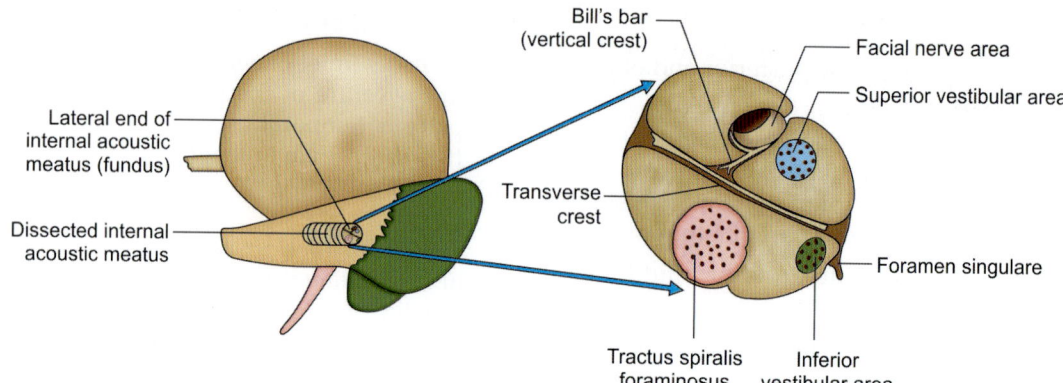

**Fig. 7.3:** Fundus of right internal acoustic meatus

## APPLIED ANATOMY

1. Thickenings of bones in the base of skull form strengthening buttresses of the skull and exert a direct effect on the pattern of fracture. Fracture lines avoid the thickenings and pass through the line of least resistance. Therefore, fractures are often zig-zag in appearance and for the same reason fracture lines often converge towards the foramen magnum or sella turcica.

2. In cases of basal fractures, laceration of structures passing through basal foramina may complicate the issue, e.g. fracture line passing through the foramen lacerum may tear the internal carotid artery with a resultant *caroticocavernous fistula* which produces *pulsating exophthalmos*.

3. If the fissure lines involve the grooves having meningeal vessels and dural sinuses, then *epidural haematoma* might result.

4. Basal fractures involving anterior cranial fossa might lead to communication between nasal cavity and subarachnoid space resulting into CSF leak into the nose. This condition is called *CSF rhinorrhoea*.

5. Fracture of tegmen tympani might connect the subarachnoid space with middle ear leading to CSF leakage into the middle ear. If the tympanic membrane is also damaged then the CSF will appear as discharge through external acoustic meatus. This condition is called *CSF otorrhoea*.

6. Communications between cranial cavity and nasal and middle ear cavities due to basal fractures may act as portal for sepsis of meninges and brain.

7. Fracture of orbital plate of frontal bone causes haemorrhage into the orbit. This haemorrhage acquires a triangular shape under the conjunctiva whose apex is towards the corneoscleral junction and base towards the orbital margin, but the exact peripheral limit of the base is not visible (Fig. 7.4).

8. Petrous temporal is very strong and therefore most fracture lines end here

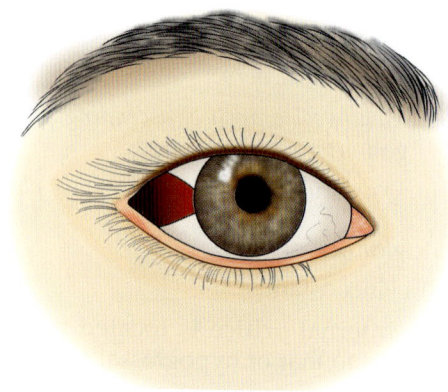

**Fig. 7.4:** Haemorrhage in the orbit

without making a tear in it. A bullet entering the middle cranial fossa through orbit, is prevented from entering the posterior cranial fossa due to the same reason.

9. A forceful hit on the forehead causes linear fracture of both vertex and base (Fig. 7.5).

10. Clinical signs and symptoms which support the involvement of base of skull, are as follows:

 i. *CSF otorrhoea* (discharge of CSF from ear).

 ii. *Tear of tympanic membrane.*

 iii. *Collection of blood in the middle ear.*

 iv. *Discolouration and edema of tissue of mastoid process* (it is due to sigmoid sinus damage).

 v. *CSF rhinorrhoea* (this is due to damage of cribriform plate).

 vi. *Cranial nerve damage* (it is due to involvement of foramina).

11. A fracture near the sella turcica may tear the stalk of pituitary gland with resulting *diabetes insipidus, impotence* and *amenorrhoea.*

12. A fracture of sphenoid may lacerate the optic nerve in optic canal resulting into blindness.

13. Fracture of cribriform plate may damage the filaments of olfactory nerve and result into *anosmia* (loss of smell sensation).

14. Petrous fracture often leads to *facial paralysis* if the facial nerve is damaged and *vertigo* and *nystagmus* if the 8th cranial nerve is involved.

15. Orbital plate of frontal bone is very important clinically:

 i. A peneterating object entering the orbit might damage its roof and then involve the frontal lobe of brain.

 ii. Orbital roof may be selected by surgeons as route to approach frontal lobe of brain.

16. A tumour in the middle cranial fossa enters the orbit through superior orbital fissure.

17. Some of the tumours which might involve the skull base are as follows:

 i. *Transitional cell carcinoma* arising from mucous membrane of paranasal sinuses or fossa of Rosenmüller of nasopharynx usually erodes the skull base.

 ii. Some of the other tumours, though very rare, arising from the base of skull or adjacent tissue are as follows: *osteomas, chondromas, chordomas, giant cell tumours of bones.*

 iii. Many malignant tumours metastasize to the basal skull bones from distant organs, e.g. prostate, lung and breast.

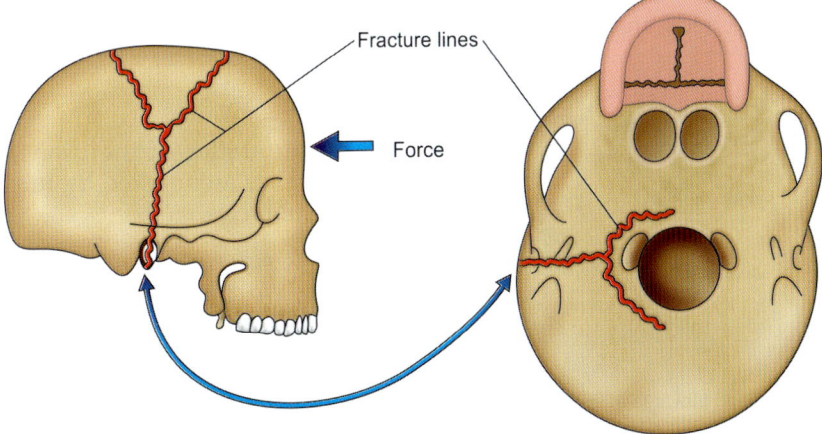

**Fig. 7.5:** Basal fracture due to blow on forehead

# 8

# Mandible

## TERMINOLOGY

The word *'mandible'* is derived from Greek word *'mandere'* which means to masticate or chew. The Latin word *'mandibula'* means lower jaw.

## PECULIARITIES (Fig. 8.1)

1. It is a 'U' shaped bone.
2. It is also called 'lower facial skeleton'.
3. Mandible is the largest and strongest bone of the face.
4. It forms the skeleton of lower jaw.

## FEATURES AND ATTACHMENTS

The mandible has a body and two rami.

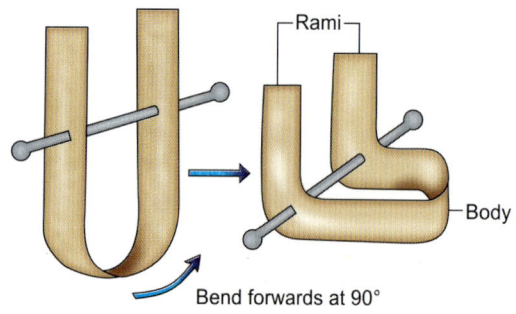

**Fig. 8.1:** Resemblance of mandible with 'U'

## I. BODY

It is shaped like a horse shoe and has 2 surfaces (external and internal) and 2 borders (upper and lower).

### A. Surfaces

### a. External surface (Figs 8.2 and 8.3)

It has following features:

### 1. Symphysis menti

It is a faint ridge on the upper part of midline indicating the fusion of two halves of mandible.

### 2. Mental protuberance

It is triangular area in the lower part of midline. The upper angle of triangle marks the lower end of symphysis menti.

### 3. Mental tubercles

The lower angles of the triangular mental protuberance are marked by tubercles called mental tubercles.

**Note:** *Remember that mental protuberance is characteristic of human jaw.*

### 4. Mental foramen

It is located below the 2nd premolar or junction between two premolar teeth. Mental nerve and vessels pass through it.

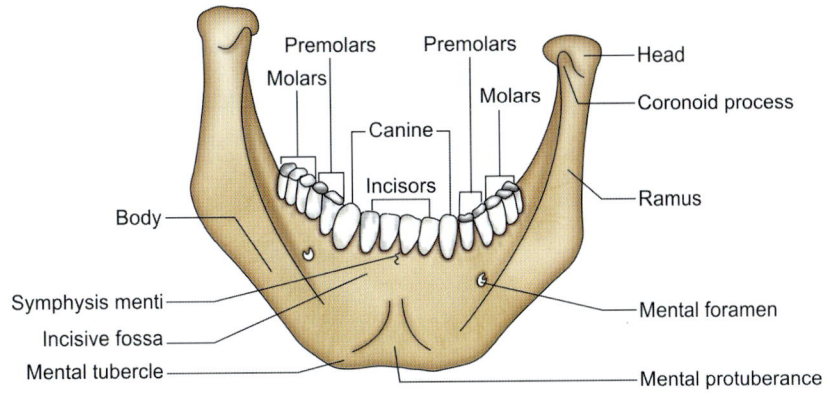

**Fig. 8.2:** Mandible: Anterior view

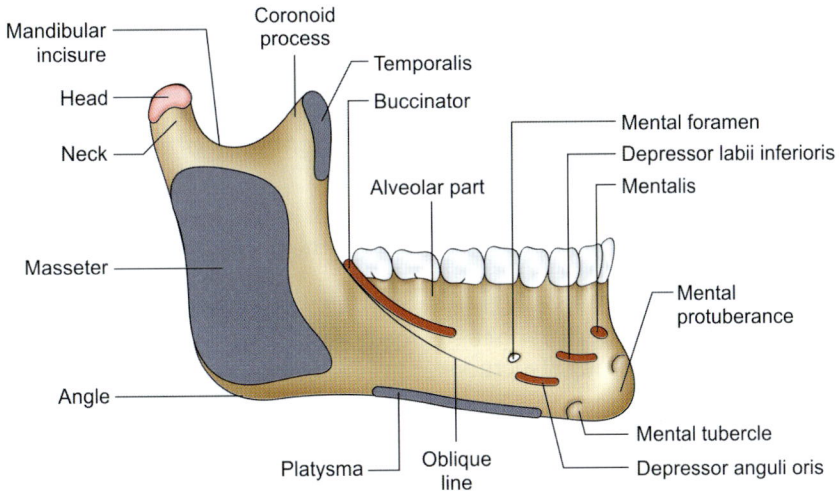

**Fig. 8.3:** Right half of mandible: External aspect

### 5. Incisive fossa

It is a shallow fossa below the incisor teeth. *Mentalis* and *orbicularis oris* originate from this fossa.

### 6. Oblique line

It is continuation of anterior border of ramus on the external surface of body. It is a faint ridge. It runs downwards and forwards to reach mental tubercle. Following muscles are attached to it from anterior to posterior:

   i. *Depressor labii inferioris.*

   ii. *Depressor anguli oris.*

   iii. *Buccinator (below the molar teeth).*

**Note:** *Junction of body and ramus is marked by the courses of facial artery and facial vein (Fig. 8.4).*

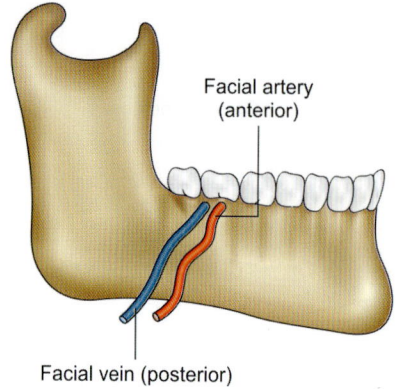

**Fig. 8.4:** Junction of body and ramus of mandible

### b. Internal surface (Figs 8.5 and 8.6)

It has following features:

#### 1. Mylohyoid line

It is an oblique ridge. It extends downwards and forwards from behind the 3rd molar tooth (1 cm below the alveolar border) to midline near the lower border between digastric fossae. *Mylohyoid muscle* is attached to it.

#### 2. Submandibular fossa

It is present below the posterior part of mylohyoid line. It lodges following structures:

    i. Submandibular salivary gland.

    ii. Facial artery.

    iii. *Submandibular lymph nodes.*

### 3. Sublingual fossa

It is an area above the anterior part of mylohyoid line. It lodges the *sublingual salivary gland.*

### 4. Genial tubercles

These are irregular elevations on either side of midline just above the anterior ends of mylohyoid lines. Upper genial tubercle provides attachment to *genioglossus muscle* while lower genial tubercle gives origin to *geniohyoid muscle.*

**Note:** *Genial tubercles are for genial muscles, since the tongue is higher as compared to the hyoid bone, the upper tubercle is for genioglossus and lower is for geniohyoid.*

### 5. Attachment of superior constrictor of pharynx

Superior constrictor originates from the area above the posterior end of mylohyoid line.

### 6. Attachment of pterygomandibular raphe

This raphe is attached to inner surface of body in continuation with the origin of superior constrictor just behind the 3rd molar tooth.

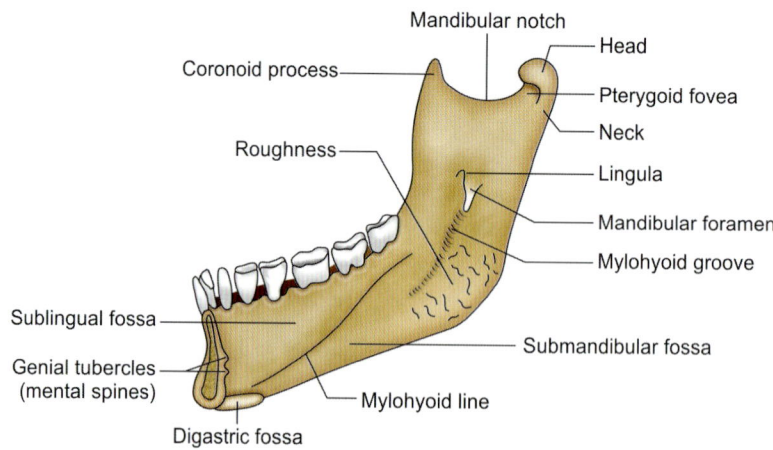

**Fig. 8.5:** Right half of mandible: Internal aspect

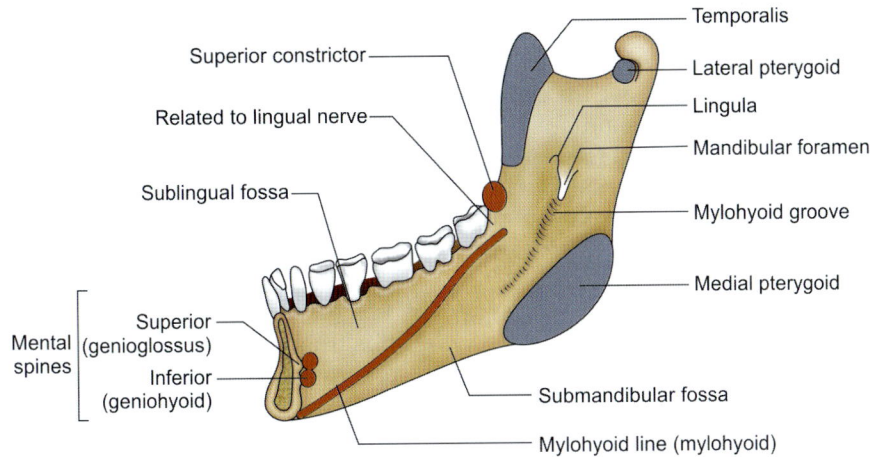

**Fig. 8.6:** Right half of mandible: Internal aspect

### 7. Relation of lingual nerve

Lingual nerve is related to mandible between the origin of superior constrictor and posterior end of mylohyoid line.

### B. Borders

#### a. Upper border (Fig. 8.7)

1. It is also called alveolar part of mandible.
2. It is hollowed out by sixteen sockets for the roots of permanent teeth.
3. The sockets vary in size and depth.
4. The sockets may be single or subdivided by septa according to the teeth which they contain.

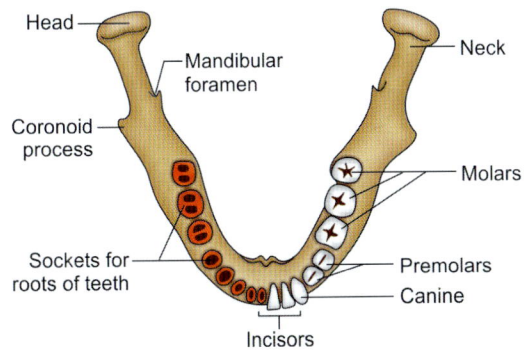

**Fig. 8.7:** Alveolar part of mandible: Superior view

#### b. Lower border

1. It is also called the *base* of mandible.
2. *Digastric fossa* is a depression at its anterior (mesial) end on each side of the midline. It receives attachment of *anterior belly of digastric.*
3. *Investing layer of deep cervical fascia* is attached to the whole length of the base.
4. *Platysma* is inserted to the lower border near the outer surface.

### II. RAMUS

Ramus of mandible has 2 surfaces (lateral and medial), 4 borders (upper, lower, anterior and posterior) and two processes (coronoid and condylar).

### A. Surfaces

#### a. Lateral surface (Fig. 8.3)

1. A small posterosuperior area is related to *parotid gland.*
2. Remaining major area provides attachment to *masseter.*

**Note:** *Remember, house of Prime Minister is located on the lateral area. P stands for Parotid and M stands for Masseter.*

## b. Medial surface (Figs 8.5 and 8.6)

1. *Mandibular foramen and canal*: Mandibular foramen is located a little above the centre of medial surface. It leads into mandibular canal which curves downwards and forwards into the body, to open on the external surface at the mental foramen. *Inferior alveolar nerve and vessels* enter the mandibular canal through the mandibular foramen.

2. *Lingula*: It is a tongue shaped projection near the anterior margin of mandibular foramen. *Sphenomandibular ligament* is attached to the lingula.

3. *Mylohyoid groove*: It begins at the lower end of mandibular foramen behind the lingula and continues downwards and forwards to reach the inner surface of body. *Mylohyoid nerve* and *vessels* occupy the mylohyoid groove.

4. Medial surface of ramus between mylohyoid groove and angle of mandible is marked by ridges. This area is meant for the attachment of *medial pterygoid*.

5. Area in front of mylohyoid groove is related to *lingual nerve*.

## B. Borders

### a. Upper border

1. It is thin.
2. It forms *mandibular notch* or *incisure*.
3. *Masseteric nerve* and *vessels* cross the mandibular notch.

### b. Lower border

1. It is backward continuation of base of mandible.
2. It meets with the posterior border of ramus to form *angle of mandible*.

### c. Anterior border

1. It is continuous above with the coronoid process and below with alveolar border of body.
2. *Temporalis* muscle is inserted on this border and adjoining medial surface.

### d. Posterior border

1. It is continuous above with the condylar process.
2. It meets with the lower border to form *angle of mandible*.
3. It is related to *parotid gland*.

## C. Processes

### a. Coronoid process

1. It is triangular upward projection from the anterosuperior part of ramus.
2. Its anterior border is continuous with the anterior border of the ramus and its posterior border bounds the mandibular notch.
3. *Temporalis muscle* gets inserted on the medial surface, apex and margins of coronoid process.

### b. Condylar process

It is an upward projection from the poterosuperior part of ramus. It consists of an upper part (*head*) and a lower part (*neck*).

#### i. Head

1. It is side to side expanded part of condylar process.
2. It articulates with the temporal bone to form *temporomandibular joint*.

#### ii. Neck

1. It is constricted part below the head.
2. It provides attachment to *capsule* in its upper part.
3. *Lateral ligament of temporomandibular joint* is attached to its lateral part.
4. *Pterygoid fovea* is a depression on its anterior aspect. *Lateral pterygoid muscle* is inserted on the pterygoid fovea.
5. Medially the neck is related to *auriculotemporal nerve* above and *maxillary artery* below.

## OSSIFICATION

1. Mandible is intramembranous as well as endochondral in origin.
2. The membrane involved is the mesenchymal sheath on the lateral aspect of both Meckel's cartilages. A centre appears on each side in this sheath during 7th week of intrauterine life.
3. Cartilages contributing to the mandible are as follows:
   i. *Anterior ends of Meckel's cartilages*
      These are invaded by bone from parent centres at 10th week of intrauterine life.
   ii. *Coronoid cartilages*
      These appear at 10th week of intrauterine life and disappear before birth.
   iii. *Condylar cartilages*
      These appear at 10th week of intrauterine life and persist till 3rd decade.
   iv. *Cartilaginous nodules*
      One or two of these nodules appear on each side of the symphysis menti at about 10th week of intrauterine life. These ossify to form mental ossicles at about the 7th month of intrauterine life and fuse with the body at the age of one year.
4. Parts of the mandible which are derived from cartilage are:

   i. Incisive part below the incisor teeth.
   ii. Coronoid and condylar processes.
   iii. Part of ramus above the mandibular foramen.

**Note:** *Remember that the names of all the parts of mandible which ossifying from cartilage start with C, i.e. coronoid process, condylar process, cranial part of ramus and chin part of body related to cutting or incisor teeth.*

5. At birth mandible consists of two halves connected at *symphysis menti.* Bony union starts from below upwards during 1st year of age and is completed at the end of 3rd year.

## AGE CHANGES IN MANDIBLE

Some of the differentiating features in different age groups are as follows:

### I. Children (Fig. 8.8)

1. The body of mandible is more like a shell having sockets for both deciduous and permanent teeth.
2. The angle of mandible measures about 140°.
3. Coronoid process is above the level of condylar process.
4. The mandibular canal and mental foramen are close to the lower border of body.

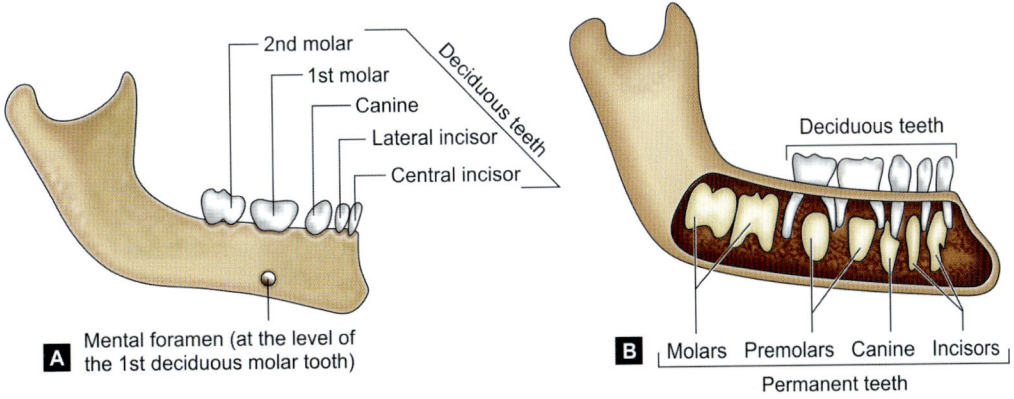

2nd molar
1st molar
Canine
Lateral incisor
Central incisor
*Deciduous teeth*

A Mental foramen (at the level of the 1st deciduous molar tooth)

Deciduous teeth

B Molars  Premolars  Canine  Incisors
Permanent teeth

**Fig. 8.8:** Right lateral view of the mandible of a child between 2 and 6 years. (A) Surface features; (B) Body dissected

## II. Adult (Fig. 8.9)

1. The alveolar and subalveolar parts of body are of equal depths.
2. The angle of mandible measures about 110°.
3. Condylar process projects above the level of coronoid process.
4. Mandibular canal runs parallel to the mylohyoid line.
5. The mental foramen is situated midway between upper and lower borders of body.

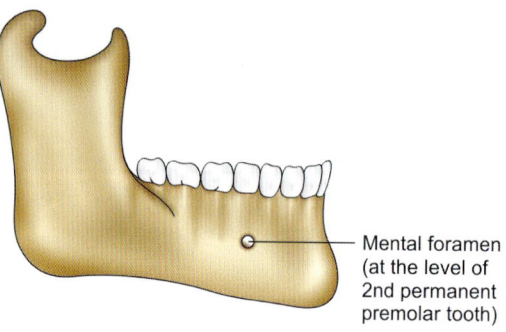

Mental foramen (at the level of 2nd permanent premolar tooth)

**Fig. 8.9:** Adult mandible: Right lateral view

## III. Old age (Fig. 8.10)

1. Loss of teeth is a usual feature.
2. Alveolar part is absorbed.
3. Angle of mandible measures about 140°
4. Neck of mandible is bent backwards making the level of coronoid process higher than condylar process.
5. Mandibular canal and mental foramen are close to the upper border of body.

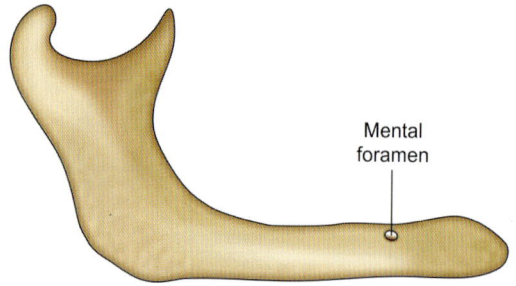

Mental foramen

**Fig. 8.10:** The mandible at old age: Right lateral view

## APPLIED ANATOMY

1. The mandible occupies a prominent and exposed position in the facial skeleton and, therefore, forms a common site of violent injuries.
2. Slender neck of the mandinble is liable to fracture as a result of violence received at the mental prominence (Fig. 8.11).

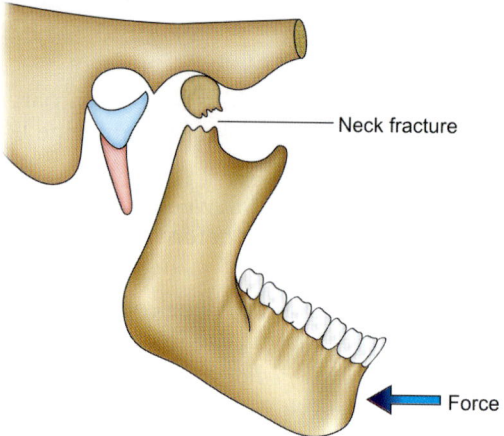

Neck fracture

Force

**Fig. 8.11:** Fracture of mandibular neck

3. Alveolar process is weaker than the rest of the mandible and, therefore, an independent alveolar fracture may occur.
4. Tendency of mandible to fracture with advancing age is due to resorption of alveolar portion of bone when the teeth are lost.
5. Elongated root of canine tooth reduces the bony substance and makes the mandible weaker at this site. Canine region is, therefore, the commonest site of fracture.
6. Thick periosteum over the mandible prevents gross displacement of fractured bones after fracture.
7. Impacted 3rd molar, mental foramen and missing teeth also contribute to the weakness in the mandible.
8. Strong muscles attached to the mandible play very important role in displacement of fractured segments of mandible. Such muscles are divided into 3 groups (Fig. 8.12).

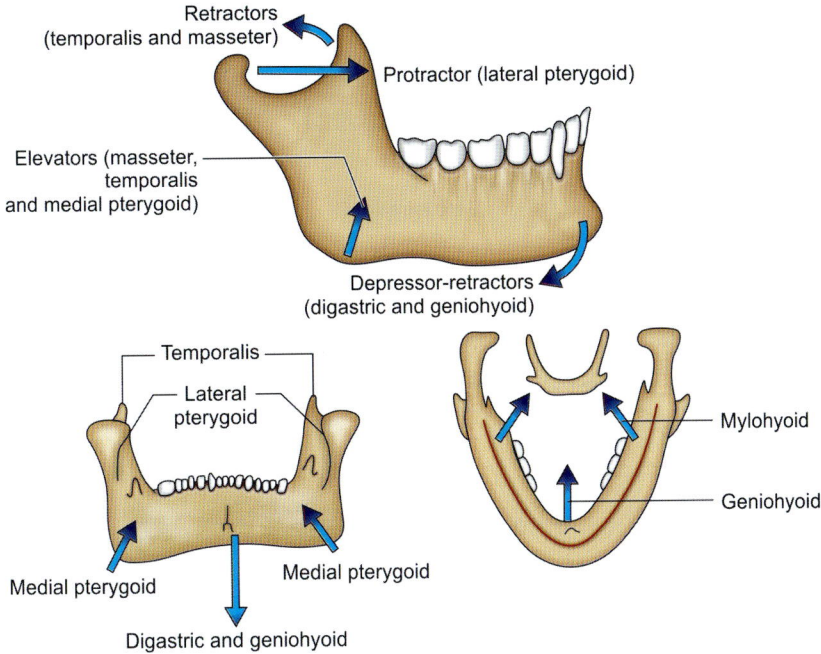

**Fig. 8.12:** Direction of composite forces of the mandibular muscles

i. *The depressor group*

It includes *geniohyoid* and *digastric muscles*. They cause posterior and inferior displacement of fractured anterior mandibular segment.

ii. *The elevator group*

The *masseter, temporalis* and *medial pterygoid muscles* belong to this group. Contraction of these muscles cause upward displacement of fractured segment if the fracture occurs in the region of angle.

iii. *The protrusor group*

It includes *lateral pterygoid muscle* which causes forward displacement of head in cases of fracture of mandibular neck.

9. Following is the general classification of mandibular fractures (Fig. 8.13):

i. *Simple*

Single fracture without exposure to exterior.

ii. *Compound*

Fractured site is exposed to exterior.

iii. *Comminuted*

It is multiple fractures of mandible at the same site. It may be both simple or compound.

iv. *Complicated*

It is fracture associated with injury of teeth, nerves or vessels.

v. *Impacted*

In this fracture one fragment has been driven into the substance of other fragment.

vi. *Greenstick*

In this fractured site bends without displacement.

vii. *Pathological*

Fracture is due to underlying diseases like osteomyelitis or tumours.

10. Clinical classification of mandibular fractures (Fig. 8.14).

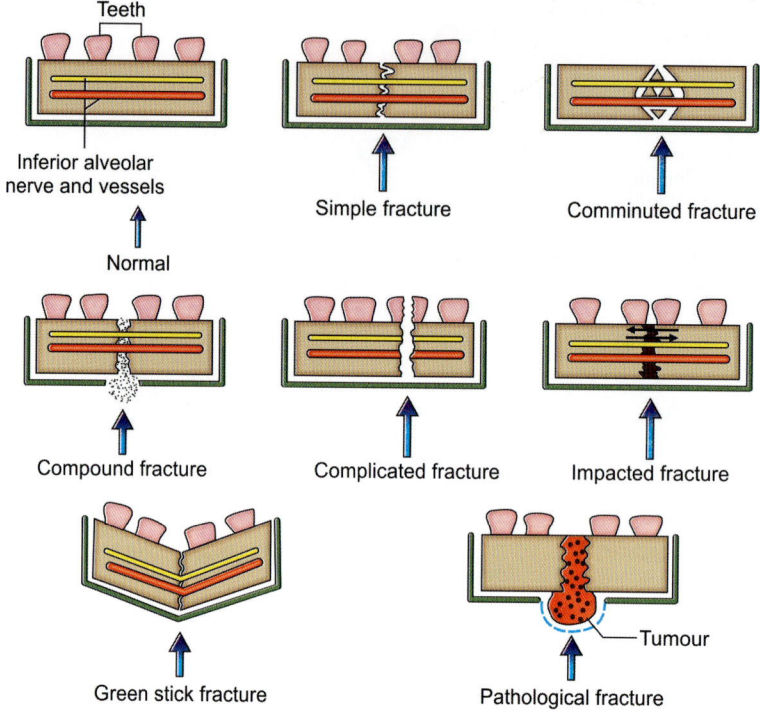

**Fig. 8.13:** Different types of fractures of mandible

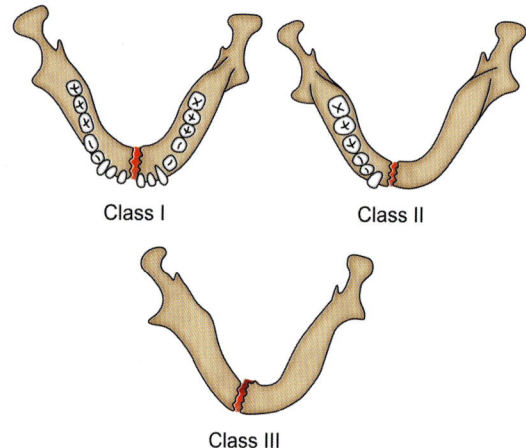

**Fig. 8.14:** Three classes of mandibular fractures

i. *Class I*

Teeth present on both sides of fractured line.

ii. *Class II*

Teeth present on one side of fractured line.

iii. *Class III*

Fragments are edentulous (without teeth)

11. Depending upon the number of sites, mandibular fractures may be of following types (Fig. 8.15):

    i. *Single unilateral*

    ii. *Double unilateral*

    iv. *Bilateral*

    v. *Multiple*

12. The mandible can be divided into following regions to simplify the sites of lesions, e.g. fractures (Fig. 8.16):

    i. *Condylar*

    ii. *Coronoid*

    iii. *Ramus*

    iv. *Angle*

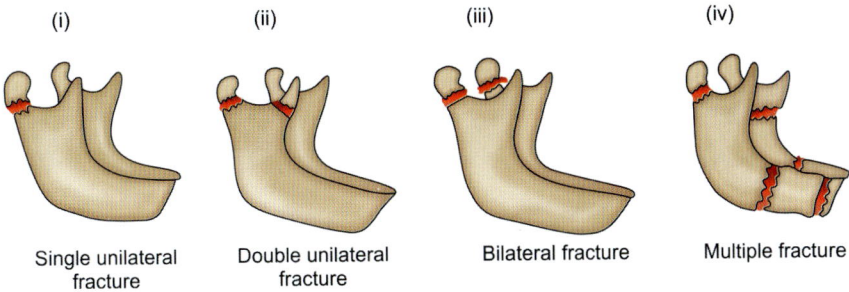

**Fig. 8.15:** Number of fractured sites as criterion for types of fractures

(i)    (ii)    (iii)    (iv)

Single unilateral fracture    Double unilateral fracture    Bilateral fracture    Multiple fracture

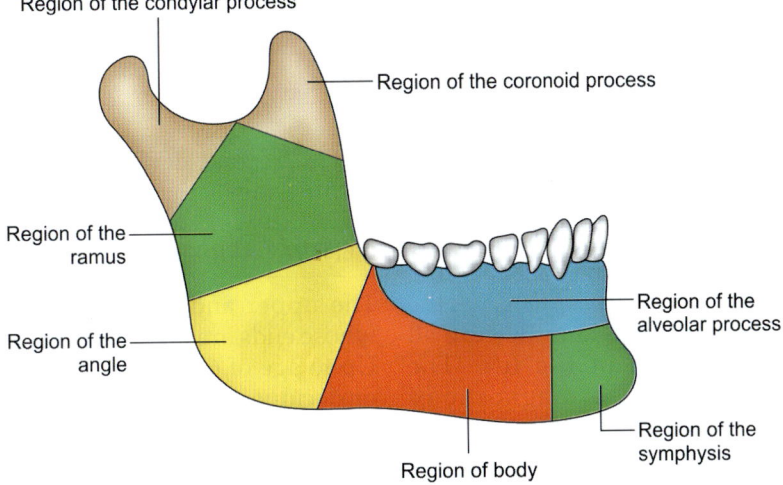

Region of the condylar process

Region of the coronoid process

Region of the ramus

Region of the angle

Region of the alveolar process

Region of body

Region of the symphysis

**Fig. 8.16:** Mandibular regions

vi. *Alveolar.*
vii. *Body.*
viii. *Symphysis.*
13. Tumours of the hard tissue of lower jaw can originate in teeth (*odontogenic tumours*) or mandible (*osteogenic tumours*)

## A. Odontogenic tumours

These can be of following two types:

### a. Odontoma

Arising from teeth proper. Odontomas may be of following three types according to their structures:

  i. *Calcified odontoma*
    It has dentine.
  ii. *Simple enamel pearl.*
    It has enamel.

  iii. *Cementoma*
    It has cementum.

### b. Ameloblastoma

Arising from the embryonal (ameloblast) cells of developing teeth.

## B. Osteogenic tumours

Following are the common osteogenic tumours:

  i. *Osteoma*
  ii. *Fibro-osteoma*
  iii. *Myxoma*
  iv. *Chondroma*
  v. *Sarcoma*
  vi. *Ewing's tumour*
  vii. *Multiple myeloma.*
  viii. *Central giant cell tumour*

# Dental Anatomy

## INTRODUCTION

In mammalian vertebrates, the teeth are constantly replaced throughout life. This condition is called *polyphyodonty*. Some mammals like rat, are *monophyodont*, i.e. the teeth are erupted once only and they are all permanent during rest of the life. The condition of *diphyodonty* is diagnostic of mammals like human being. In this condition there are two dentitions. The first dentition is called *primary* or *deciduous* because the teeth fall after a definite period like falling of the leaves. Second dentition is called *permanent* because the teeth persist throughout life.

## GENERAL ARRANGEMENT

The upper and lower jaws are like arches whose ends are directed posteriorly (Fig. 9.1). Up to age of 6 years the teeth are temporary or deciduous.

Normally there are five deciduous teeth in each half of both the jaws. These are named from anterior midpoint to posterior end on each side as follows (Fig. 9.2):

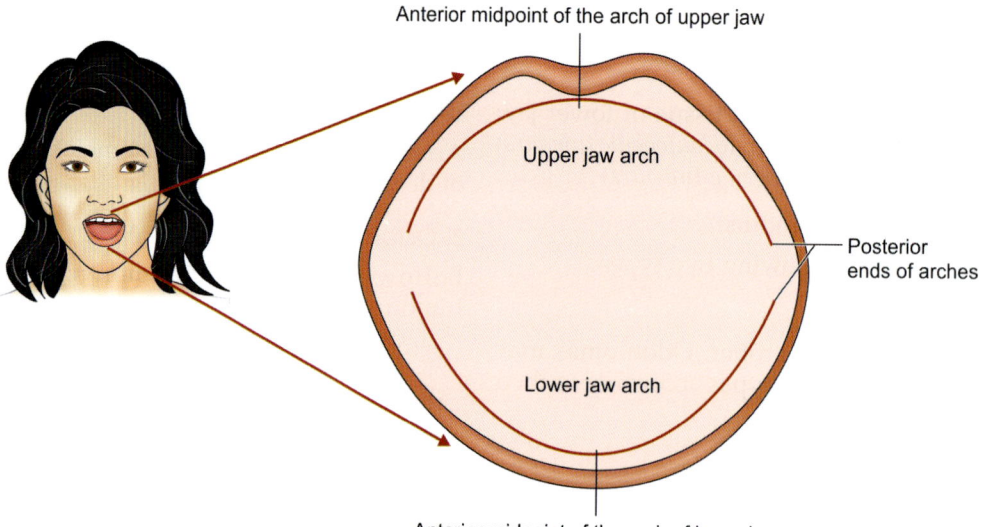

**Fig. 9.1:** Jaw arches

66

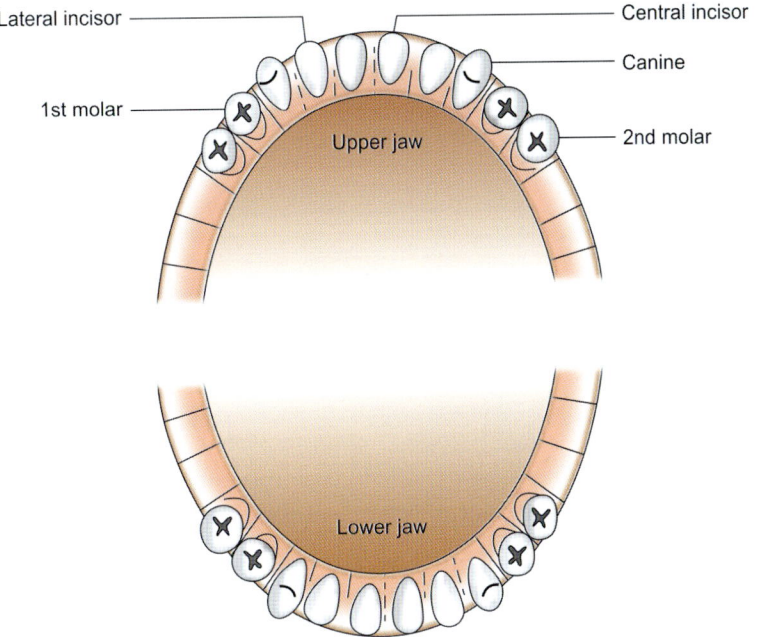

**Fig. 9.2:** Arrangement of deciduous teeth

1. *Central incisor*
2. *Lateral incisor*
3. *Canine*
4. *First molar*
5. *Second molar*

In adult the teeth are permanent in nature. Normally there are eight permanent teeth in each half of both the jaws. These are named from anterior midpoint to posterior end on each side as follows (Fig. 9.3):

1. *Central incisor*
2. *Lateral incisor*
3. *Canine*
4. *First premolar*
5. *Second premolar*
6. *First molar*
7. *Second molar*
8. *Third molar*

## DENTAL FORMULA

Deciduous teeth — 2102

$$\text{or} \quad I\frac{2}{2} C\frac{1}{1} M\frac{2}{2} = 10$$

Permanent teeth — 2123

$$\text{or} \quad I\frac{2}{2} C\frac{1}{1} P\frac{2}{2} M\frac{3}{3} = 16$$

## CLINICAL NOTATION SYSTEM

### A. Zsigmondy numbering system

#### a. Permanent teeth

Permanent dentition is identified by assigning a number of teeth from 1 through 8 with each quadrant. In this system, the number 8 represents 3rd molars whereas number 1 represents central incisors (Fig. 9.4). The quadrants are as follows:

= Maxillary right
= Maxillary left
= Mandibular left
= Mandibular right

### b. Primary teeth

The primary teeth can be identified using the same basic system. The teeth in the quadrant are labeled with letters A through E. The primary 2nd molars are assigned the letter E

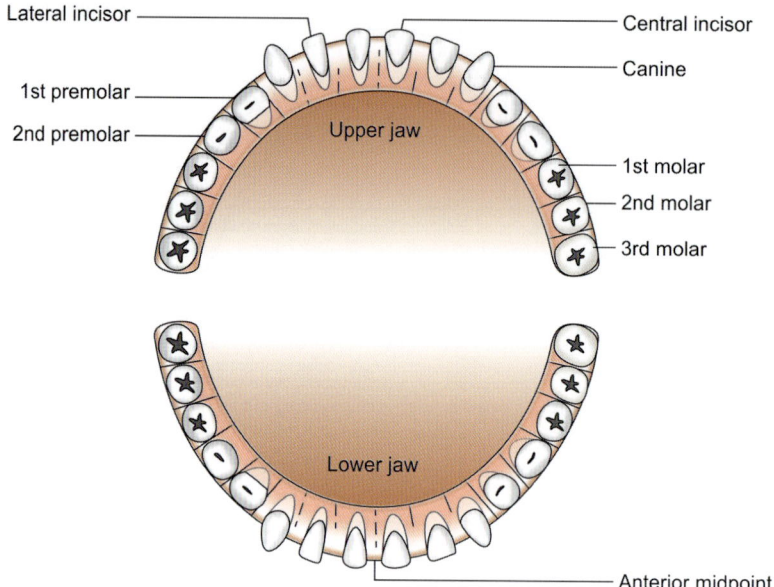

**Fig. 9.3:** Arrangement of permanent teeth

| Maxillary right | | | | | | | | Maxillary left | | | | | | | |
|---|---|---|---|---|---|---|---|---|---|---|---|---|---|---|---|
| 8 | 7 | 6 | 5 | 4 | 3 | 2 | 1 | 1 | 2 | 3 | 4 | 5 | 6 | 7 | 8 |
| 8 | 7 | 6 | 5 | 4 | 3 | 2 | 1 | 1 | 2 | 3 | 4 | 5 | 6 | 7 | 8 |
| Mandibular right | | | | | | | | Mandibular left | | | | | | | |

**Fig. 9.4:** Zsigmondy numbering system for permanent teeth

and the central incisors are assigned the letter A (Fig. 9.5).

| Maxillary right | | | | | Maxillary left | | | | |
|---|---|---|---|---|---|---|---|---|---|
| E | D | C | B | A | A | B | C | D | E |
| E | D | C | B | A | A | B | C | D | E |
| Mandibular right | | | | | Mandibular left | | | | |

**Fig. 9.5:** Zsigmondy numbering system for primary teeth

## B. FDI (Federation Dentaire Internationale) tooth numbering system

This system uses a two digit number to identify each tooth. The first digit indicates the quadrant in which the tooth is located. The 2nd digit identifies the specific tooth in that quadrant (Fig. 9.6). The quadrants for permanent teeth are numbered as follows:

Quadrant No. 1 = Maxillary right
Quadrant No. 2 = Maxillary left
Quadrant No. 3 = Mandibular left
Quadrant No. 4 = Mandibular right

*The quardrants in primary dentition are numbered as follows (Fig. 9.7):*

Quadrant No. 5 = Maxillary right
Quadrant No. 6 = Maxillary left
Quadrant No. 7 = Mandibular left
Quadrant No. 8 = Mandibular right

## C. ADA (American Dental Association) sequential numbering system.

The ADA has adopted a standard sequential numbering system for all 32 teeth in the permanent dentition. Each tooth is assigned

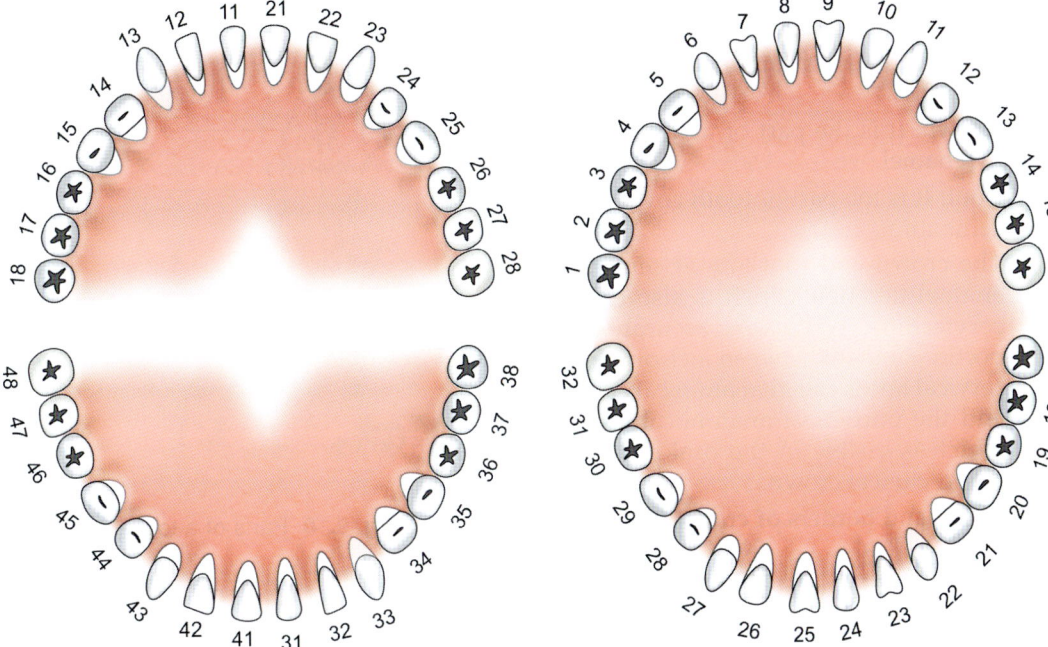

**Fig. 9.6:** FDI tooth numbering system for permanent dentition

**Fig. 9.8:** ADA sequential numbering system of permanent dentition

ADA system can also be used to identify the primary teeth except that they are identified with letters A through T (Fig. 9.9).

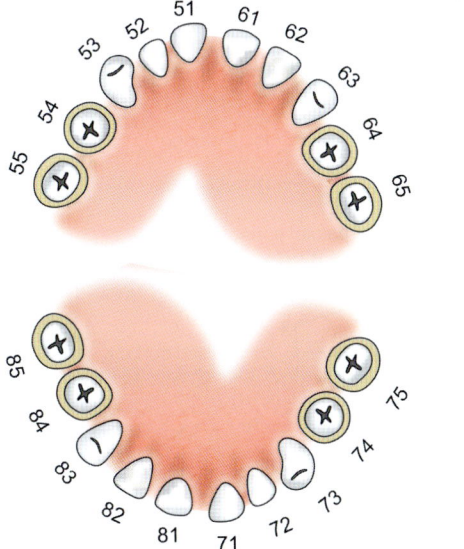

**Fig. 9.7:** FDI numbering system for primary dentition

a number so that whenever that number is used it will indicate a specific permanent tooth (Fig. 9.8).

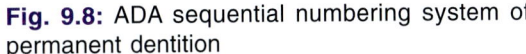

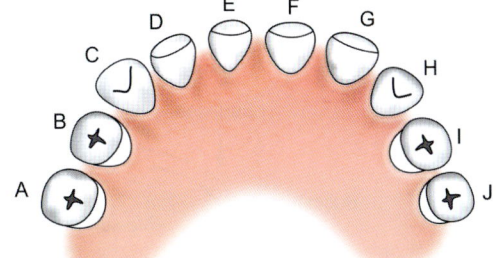

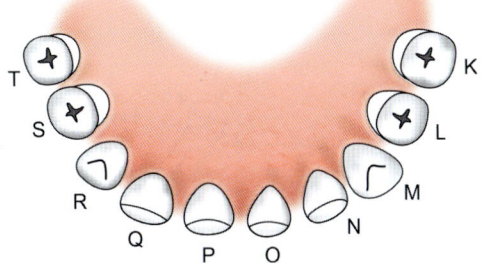

**Fig. 9.9:** ADA system for numbering primary teeth

## MORPHOLOGY OF PERMANENT TEETH

**A. Parts:** Each tooth is comprised of 2 parts (Fig. 9.10):

  1. **Crown:** It is the part of tooth covered by enamel.

  2. **Root:** It is the part of tooth covered by cementum.

  The crown and root join at cemento-enamel junction which is also called cervicalline. To be very accurate, the portion of tooth between incisor line to cervical line is called anatomical crown and the portion of anatomical crown which is visible in the oral cavity is called clinical crown.

**B. Surfaces and borders of crown** (Fig. 9.11)

  a. Incisor

  It has an incisal edge and four surfaces:

    1. *Labial (outer)*
    2. *Lingual or palatal (inner)*
    3. *Mesial (medial)*
    4. *Distal (lateral)*

  b. Canine

  It has single cusp (instead of incisal edge of incisor) and four surfaces (like incisors)

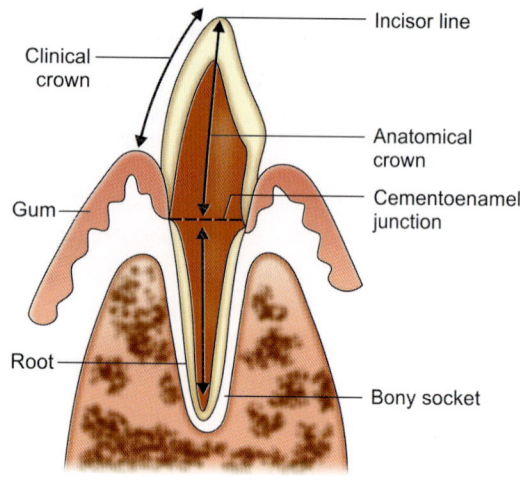

**Fig. 9.10:** Parts of a tooth

  c. Premolar and molar

  These have five surfaces:

    1. *Occlusal*
    2. *Buccal*
    3. *Lingual or palatal*
    4. *Mesial*
    5. *Distal*

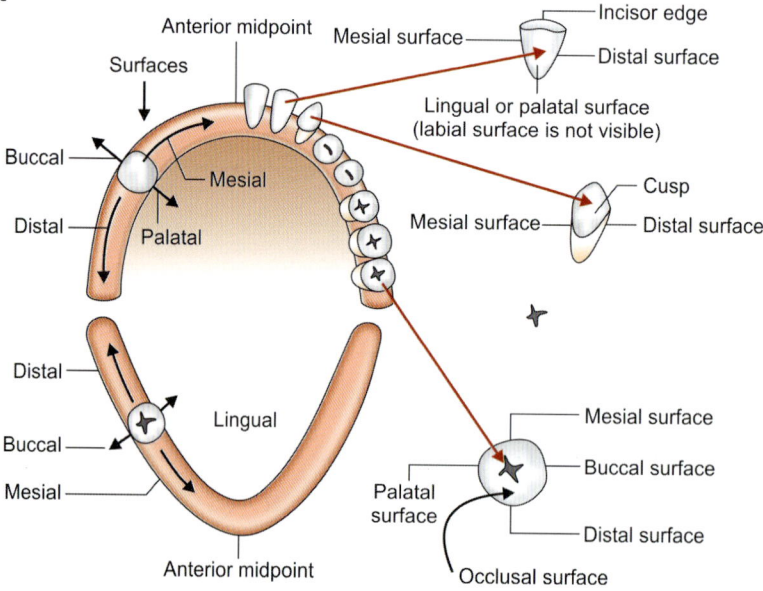

**Fig. 9.11:** Surfaces and borders of crown

## C. Cusps of the crowns of permanent teeth

Cusps are miniature tubercles on the occlusal surface of crown (Fig. 9.12). There is no cusp in incisor tooth. Canine has got single cusp and, therefore, is also called *cuspid tooth*. Premolar has two cusps (buccal and palatal) and, therefore, is also called *bicuspid tooth*.

Upper molars have usually four cusps:

1. *Mesio-palatal*

2. *Mesio-buccal*

3. *Disto-palatal*

4. *Disto-buccal*

Lower (mandibular) 1st molar has usually five cusps:

1. *Mesio-lingual*

2. *Mesio-buccal*

3. *Disto-lingual*

4. *Disto-buccal*

5. *Distal*

Lower 2nd molar has generally four cusps like upper molars. Mandibular 3rd molar shows irregular development of crown portion.

## D. Roots of permanent teeth

Incisors, canine and premolars have usually one root each, except upper 1st premolar which has two roots (buccal and palatal). Upper molars have three roots, of which two are buccal (one mesial and another distal) and one is palatal. The lower molars have usually two roots (one mesial and another distal) (Fig. 9.13).

## DIFFERENCES BETWEEN PERMANENT AND PRIMARY TEETH

1. Primary teeth are usually lighter in colour than the permanent teeth.

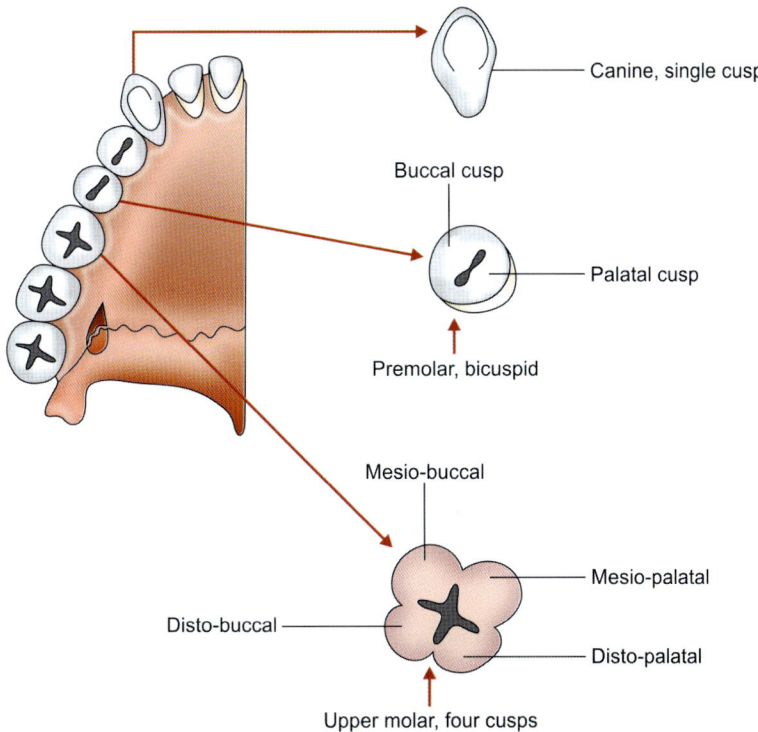

Canine, single cusp

Buccal cusp

Palatal cusp

Premolar, bicuspid

Mesio-buccal

Mesio-palatal

Disto-buccal

Disto-palatal

Upper molar, four cusps

**Fig. 9.12:** Cusps of the crown

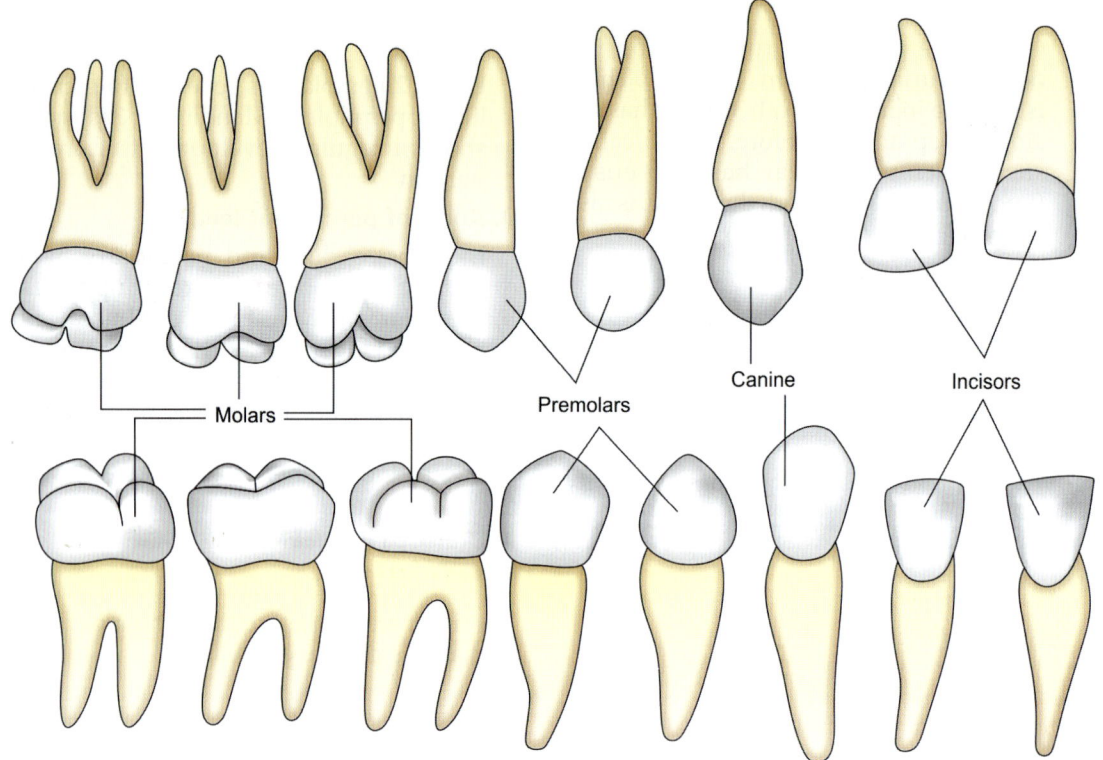

**Fig. 9.13:** Right sided permanent teeth: Buccal view

2. Primary anterior teeth are smaller than their permanent successors in both crown and root portions.
3. Primary molars are wider mesiodistally than the permanent premolars that replace them.
4. Roots of primary molars diverge to accommodate the permanent premolars.
5. Roots of primary teeth are longer than those of permanent teeth compared to crown length.
6. Buccal and lingual surfaces of crowns of primary molars taper occlusally than do the permanent molars.
7. In primary teeth the pulp chambers are relatively larger than those in permanent teeth when compared with the crown.
8. Enamel in primary teeth is relatively thin.

## ERUPTION OF TEETH

All the teeth erupt after birth. The deciduous teeth start appearing at the six months of age and continue erupting up to two years (Fig. 9.14). Permanent tooth is first seen at the age of 6 years. Eruption of all the permanent teeth is completed by the end of twelve years except third molars which appear between 18 and 25 years.

## FUNCTIONS OF TEETH

1. Incisors are cutting teeth and, therefore, these are chisel like.
2. Canine is conical in shape and is meant for tearing. Canine teeth are well developed in carnivores.

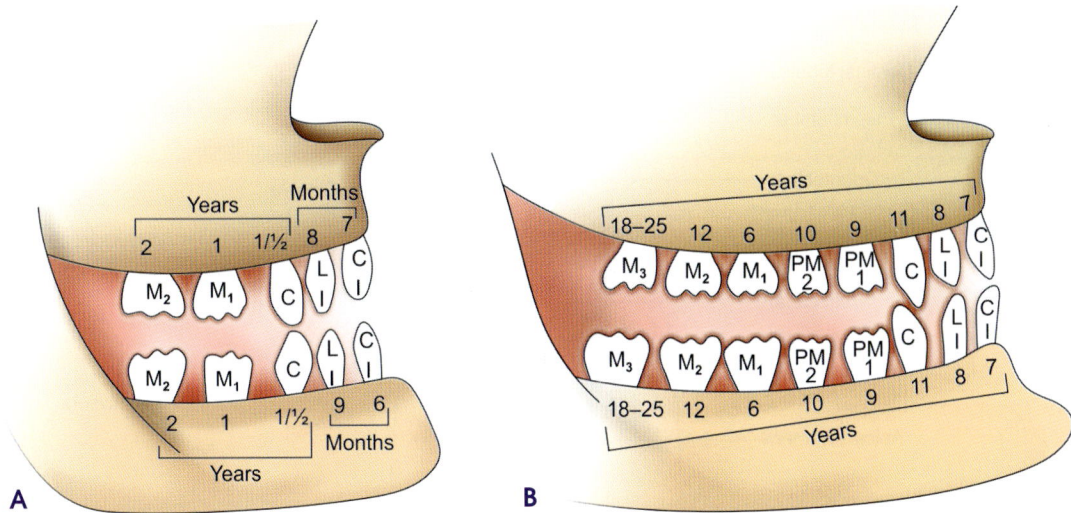

**Fig. 9.14:** Times of eruption of teeth: (A) Primary dentition and (B) Permanent dentition

3. Molars are grinding teeth and, therefore, have cusps on their occlusal surfaces.
4. Maxillary molars assist the mandibular molars in performing the major portion of the work in the mastication and comminution of food.

## STRUCTURE OF TOOTH

1. Hard part of the tooth is made up of three types of bones:
   i. *Dentine*
   ii. *Enamel*
   iii. *Cement*
2. The tooth is traversed by a cavity called pulp cavity.
3. Pulp cavity is lined by odontoblasts and contains vascular connective tissue and sensory nerve fibres.
4. Dentine resembles bone but is harder and without lacunae and bone cells. It consists of diverging dentinal tubules containing fibres (of *Tomes*) of the odontoblast cells (Fig. 9.15).
5. Substance immediately surrounding the tubule is relatively thicker forming dentinal (*Neumann's*) sheath.

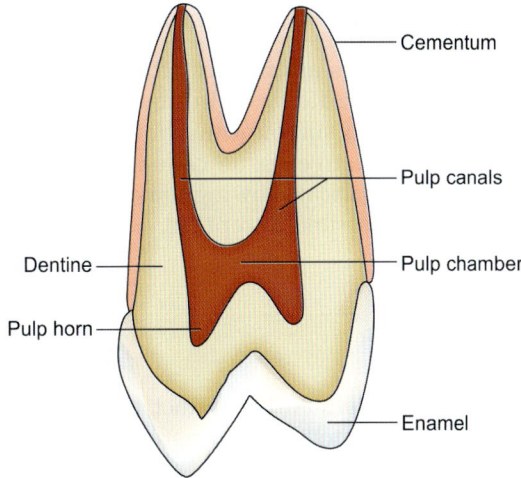

**Fig. 9.15:** Subdivision of the pulp cavity of a tooth

6. Enamel covers the dentine of crown. Enamel is the hardest substance in the body and composed of 90% inorganic salts such as calcium phosphate and carbonate. It consists of elongated enamel rods or prisms.
7. Cement covers the dentine of the root. It is similar to bone in structure having bone cells (Fig. 9.16).

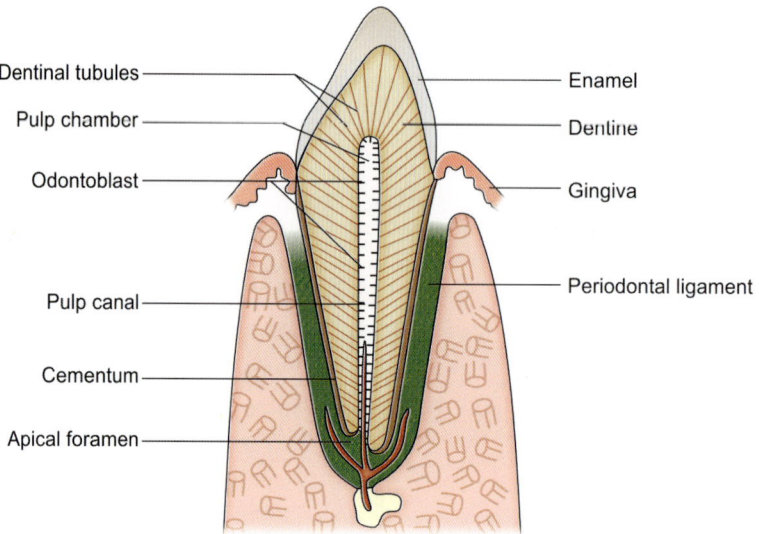

**Fig. 9.16:** Structure of the tooth

## ATTACHMENT OF TOOTH WITH JAW

Teeth of reptiles are rigidly attached to the jaw bone by hard *cement*. In mammals teeth are attached to surrounding bone tissue of jaw by connective tissue called *periodontal membrane* or *ligament* allowing some movement which is impossible in reptiles.

## OCCLUSION

### A. Definition

Occlusion is defined as contact relationship of the teeth in function and parafunction.

### B. Position of teeth

  a. Premolars and molars

    In occlusion the buccal cusps of the lower cheek teeth lie between buccal and palatal cusps of the upper cheek teeth. At the same time the lower cheek tooth is slightly in front of the corresponding upper cheek tooth. In other words the lower cheek tooth is slightly lingual and measial to the corresponding upper cheek tooth (Fig. 9.17).

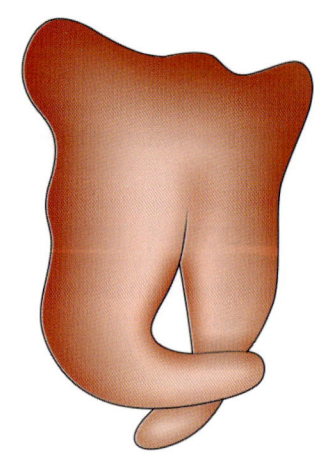

**Fig. 9.17:** Occlusal position of premolar and molar teeth

  b. Canine

    During occlusion, the lower canine is in front of upper canine.

  c. Incisors

    When the teeth are clinched (position of occlusion), the lingual surface of the upper incisor normally obscures the upper 1/3rd of the labial surface of the lower incisor.

## APPLIED ANATOMY

1. Tooth is the hardest and most stable tissue of the body and therefore can be fossilized and preserved for medicolegal purpose or study of evolution.

2. Temporary ridges on the teeth represent localized disturbances of calcification in developing teeth and may be correlated with diseases.

3. Use of tetracycline should be avoided during 3rd trimester to 12 years of age as it stains the teeth.

4. The normal location of 1st molar is at the centre of the fully developed adult jaw anteroposteriorly. Due to this significant position, the 1st molar is considered the corner stone of dental arches.

5. The stability of occlusion and maintenance of tooth position are dependent upon all of the forces that act upon the teeth. Occlusive forces, eruptive forces, lip and cheek pressure and tongue pressure are all involved in maintaining the position of teeth.

6. Eruption of the teeth is retarded in cases of vitamin deficiency.

7. Distortion of roots may be an associated feature in *cleido-cranial dysostosis*, a hereditary disorder (Fig. 9.18).

8. There may be discolouration of tooth in some diseases. Darkish brown teeth are marked in cases of *osteogenesis imperfecta*.

9. Early eruption of deciduous dentition is usually hereditary but the retarted eruption are observed in diseases like *cretinism* and *rickets*.

10. Impaction of the mandibular 3rd molar occurs most frequently.

11. Anomalies in number of teeth:

Complete developmental absence of teeth is called *anodontia*. It is a rare condition. Additional teeth (*supernumerary teeth*) are relatively more frequent.

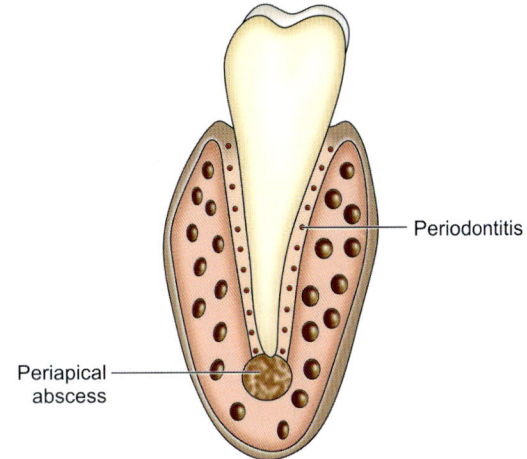

Periodontitis

Periapical abscess

**Fig. 9.18:** Distortion of roots in cleidocranial dysostosis

12. Abnormalities in size of teeth:

*Megadontia* and *microdontia* are the terms used to denote teeth that are unusually large and small respectively.

13. *Mottling* or irregular patches of white or brownish pigmentation of the teeth are associated with small amount of fluoride in the drinking water. Since the accurence is world wide, though only in certain regions of each country, the condition is called *endemic fluorosis*.

14. *Dental caries*, a very common destructive lesion of tooth, is due to dissolution of dental tissue by microbially produced acids.

15. *Pulpitis*

Inflammation of pulp of the tooth is called pulpitis. Dental caries is the most frequent factor in producing inflammatory change in pulp.

16. *Periodontitis*

It is an inflammation of the membrane surrounding the root of tooth (Fig. 9.19). When single tooth is involved, the condition is called 'local periodontitis'. In 'general periodontitis', several teeth are involved.

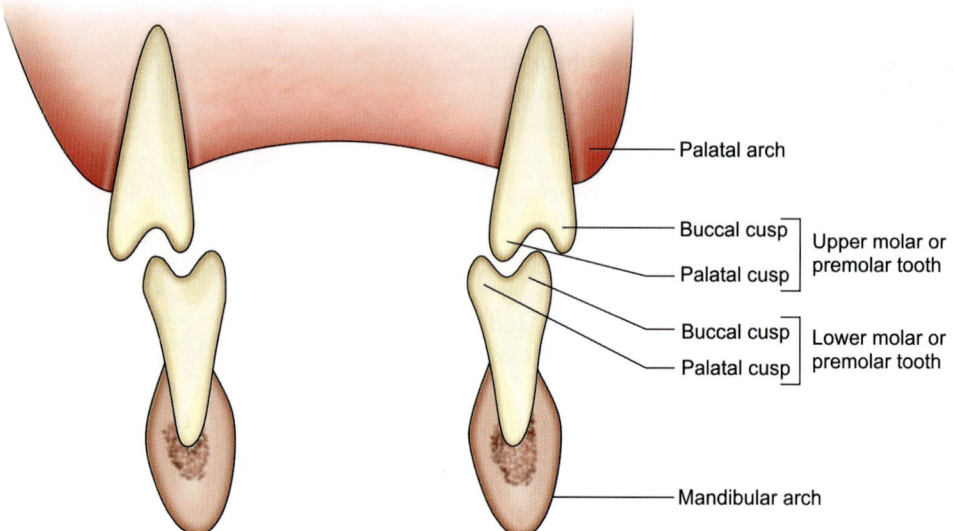

Palatal arch

Buccal cusp  ⎤ Upper molar or
Palatal cusp ⎦ premolar tooth

Buccal cusp  ⎤ Lower molar or
Palatal cusp ⎦ premolar tooth

Mandibular arch

**Fig. 9.19:** Periodontitis and periapical abscess

17. *Periapical abscess*

    Periodontitis in the region of apex of tooth may lead to pus formation, a condition known as periapical abscess.

18. Teeth are often the sites of cysts (*odontogenic cysts*) or tumours (*odontogenic tumours*).

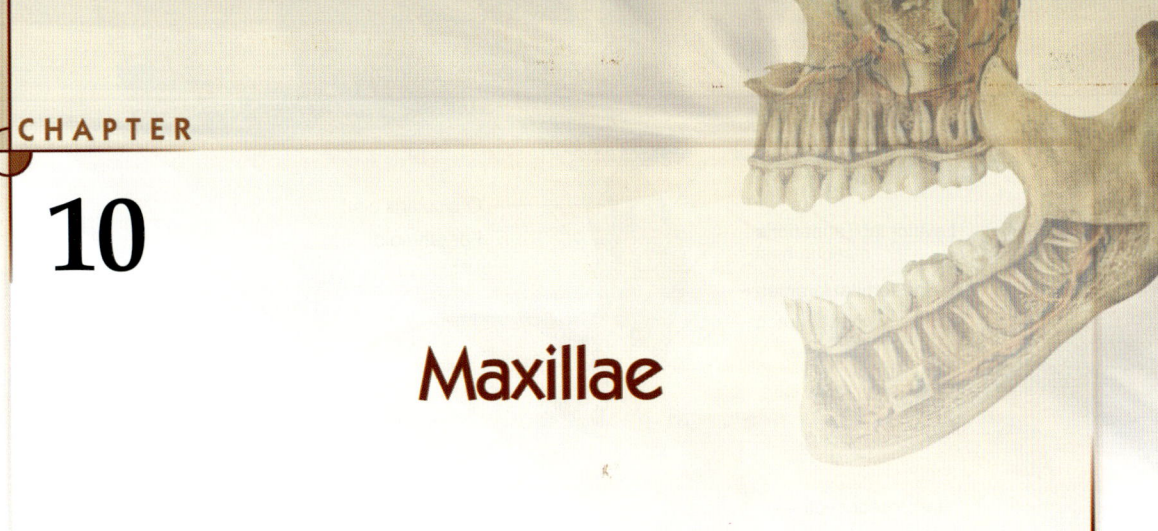

# 10

# Maxillae

## TERMINOLOGY

Maxilla is a Latin word meaning 'cheek' or 'jaw'. The word is commonly used in reference to upper jaw.

## LOCATION

1. There are two maxillae which form major part of upper facial skeleton.
2. Whole of the upper jaw is formed by two maxillae.
3. Junction of two maxillae is marked by intermaxillary suture visible in the hard palate and face in midline.

## FEATURES AND ATTACHMENTS

Each maxilla consists of a body and four processes (zygomatic, frontal, alveolar and palatine).

## I. BODY (Figs 10.1 and 10.2)

It has four surfaces (anterior, infratemporal, orbital and nasal).

### A. Anterior surface

1. It is directed forwards and laterally.
2. There is a vertical elevation at the site of socket for canine root. This is called *canine eminence*.

3. Medial to canine eminence is a depression called *incisive fossa* which gives origin to *depressor septi*.
4. The anterior surface below the incisive fossa gives attachments to *incisivus superior* and *orbicularis oris*.
5. Just above the incisive fossa there is attachment of *nasalis muscle.*
6. Lateral to canine eminence is another fossa called *canine fossa. Levator anguli oris* originates from the canine fossa.
7. Above the canine fossa is a foramen called *infraorbital foramen*. It transmits *infraorbital nerve and vessels.*
8. Above the infra-orbital foramen is sharp infra-orbital margin which gives origin to *levator labii superioris.*
9. Its upper part is limited medially by a deep notch called *nasal notch.*

### B. Infratemporal surface

1. It faces backwards and laterally.
2. It forms anterior wall of *infratemporal fossa.*
3. It shows 2–3 openings of *alveolar canals* which transmit *posterior superior alveolar nerves and vessels.*
4. Its inferoposterior part is marked by *maxillary tuberosity* which articulates with the pyramidal process of palatine bone.

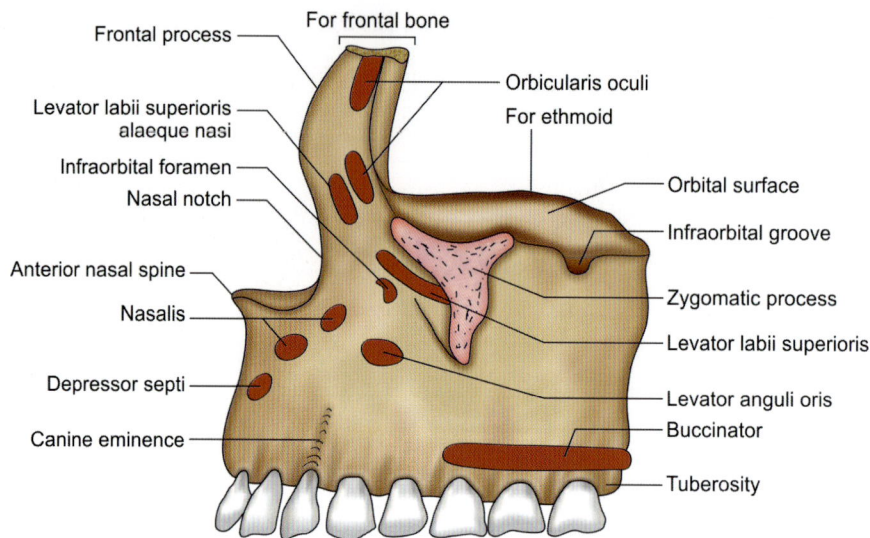

**Fig. 10.1:** Left maxilla: Lateral aspect

### C. Orbital surface

1. It forms floor of orbit.

2. Running forwards is *infraorbital groove* in the middle of its posterior part. The groove continues with *infra-orbital canal* which opens on the anterior surface as *infraorbital foramen.* It is meant for *infraorbital nerve and vessels.*

3. Anteromedially it gives origin to *inferior oblique muscle.*

4. It has three borders (medial, posterior and anterior).

#### a. Medial border

It is marked anteriorly by *lacrimal notch.* Behind this notch this border provides attachments to lacrimal bone, orbital plate of ethmoid and orbital process of palatine bone from before backwards.

#### b. Posterior border

It forms anterior border of inferior orbital fissure.

#### c. Anterior border

It contributes to the medial part of infra-orbital margin.

### D. Nasal surface (Fig. 10.2)

1. It forms the lateral wall of nasal cavity.

2. A large opening (*maxillary hiatus*) is the most prominent feature of this surface.

3. Maxillary hiatus leads into *maxillary sinus,* a large air space within the body of maxilla.

4. Maxillary hiatus is greatly reduced in size in articulated skull by ethmoid (uncinate process) and lacrimal bone above, inferior concha below and perpendicular plate of palatine bone behind.

5. Below the hiatus this surface forms inferior meatus of nasal cavity.

6. Posterior part of nasal surface has got an *oblique groove* which is converted into *greater palatine canal* by perpendicular plate of palatine bone. Greater palatine nerve and vessels pass through this canal.

7. In front of hiatus is *nasolacrimal groove*. This is converted into *nasolacrimal canal* by lacrimal bone and inferior concha. This canal is meant for *nasolacrimal duct.*

8. An oblique ridge called *conchal crest,* is present in front of nasolacrimal groove. It articulates with inferior concha.

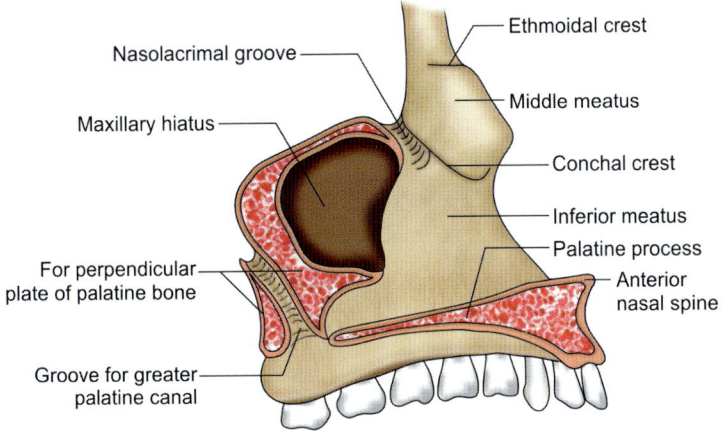

**Fig. 10.2:** Left maxilla: Medial aspect

## II. PROCESSES

### A. Zygomatic process

It has three surfaces, anterior, posterior and superior. The latter is rough for articulation with zygomatic bone.

### B. Frontal process

It possesses an upper end, two surfaces (lateral and medial) and two borders (anterior and posterior).

#### a. Upper end

It articulates with the nasal notch of frontal bone.

#### b. Surfaces

##### i. Lateral surface (Fig. 10.1)

1. It has a vertical ridge (*anterior lacrimal crest*) in the middle for the attachment of *medial palpebral ligament*.
2. Area in front of crest gives attachments to *orbicularis oculi* and *levator labii superioris alaeque nasi*.
3. Area behind the lacrimal crest contributes to the anterior half of lacrimal groove.

##### ii. Medial surface (Fig. 10.2)

1. It has got a horizontal ridge (*ethmoidal crest*) in its middle. It articulates with middle nasal concha.
2. A roughened area above the crest articulates with ethmoid to complete anterior ethmoidal air cells.
3. The area below the ethmoidal crest forms *atrium* of middle meatus.

#### c. Borders

##### i. Anterior border

It articulates with nasal bone.

##### ii. Posterior border

It articulates with lacrimal bone.

### C. Alveolar process

1. It is arched lower border of body.
2. It has sockets for upper teeth.
3. *Buccinator* originates from the posterior part of outer surface over the sockets for permanent molars roots.

### D. Palatine process

It is a horizontal bracket like projection from the lower part of medial surface of body. It forms anterior 3/4th of hard palate. It has two surfaces (superior and inferior) and three borders (medial, posterior and lateral).

### a. Surfaces

#### i. Superior surface

1. It is concave and smooth.
2. It forms floor of nasal cavity.

#### ii. Inferior surface

1. It has *depressions* for palatine glands.
2. It has several *nutrient foramina* for nutrient vessels.
3. *Greater palatine groove* for greater palatine nerve and vessels is present in its posterolateral part.
4. When two maxillae meet, *incisive fossa* is noticed behind the incisor teeth.
5. *Incisive canal* is communication between incisive fossa and nasal cavity. It transmits *greater palatine artery* and *nasopalatine nerve*.

### b. Borders

#### i. Medial border

1. It meets with the similar border of opposite maxilla to form *intermaxillary suture*.
2. This border is raised into a ridge called *nasal crest*. Nasal crests of two sides enclose a groove to receive the vomer.
3. Its anterior end is prolonged and meets with the similar prolongation of opposite side to form *anterior nasal spine*.

#### ii. Posterior border

It articulates with the anterior border of horizontal plate of palatine bone to form *palatomaxillary suture*.

#### iii. Lateral border

It fuses with the body.

### OSSIFICATION

1. The maxilla is intramembranous in origin.
2. It develops in the mesenchyme just superficial to nasal capsule.

3. Three centres of ossification appear:
   i. One centre appears for the main mass just above canine fossa at about 6th week of intrauterine life.
   ii. Two centres appear for os incisivum (premaxillary part).

**Note:** *Remember that premaxilla is that part of maxilla which holds incisor teeth and is a separate bone in most mammalian upper jaws.*

4. Maxillary sinus appears on the nasal aspect as a groove at about 4th month of intrauterine life.

### AGE CHANGES IN MAXILLA

#### I. At birth

1. Vertical diameter is lesser than both the transverse and anteroposterior diameters.
2. Body is mainly occupied by sockets for the teeth.
3. Maxillary sinus is seen as a shallow groove on the nasal aspect.

#### II. Adult

1. Vertical diameter is greater than the transverse and anteroposterior diameters.
2. Maxillary sinus has greatly developed within the body.

#### III. Old age

1. Due to falling of teeth and resorption of alveolar margin, the vertical diameter is again greatly reduced.
2. Alveolar margin is reduced in thickness at the expense of the labial wall.

### APPLIED ANATOMY

**1. Maxillary sinus (antrum of Highmore)**

It is the air space in the body of maxilla. It is pyramidal in shape with base towards nasal cavity and apex towards zygomatic process. Its height and anteroposterior measurements are 1.5 inches each while width is 1 inch only. It is very important clinically due to following facts:

i. It is largest paranasal sinus and commonly involved during inflammation process (maxillary sinusitis).

ii. It drains into middle meatus which is higher than its floor. The latter is about 1.25 cm below the floor of nasal cavity. To facilitate the drainage of pus in maxillary sinus an opening is made in inferior meatus by operative procedures like *antral puncture* or *antrostomy* (Fig. 10.3).

iii. *Maxillary tumours* can produce a bulging in adjacent related surroundings, i.e. superiorly in the floor of orbit, inferiorly in the roof of oral cavity, anteriorly in the face, posteriorly in the infratemporal fossa and medially in the lateral wall of nasal cavity.

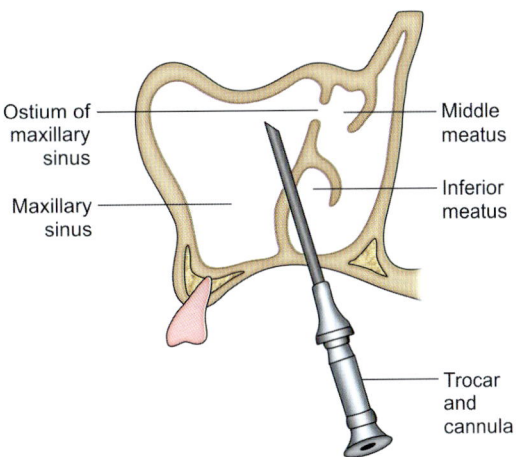

**Fig. 10.3:** Antral puncture

**2. Maxillary fractures (Fig. 10.4)**

A. Unilateral fracture of maxilla usually involves its alveolar process.

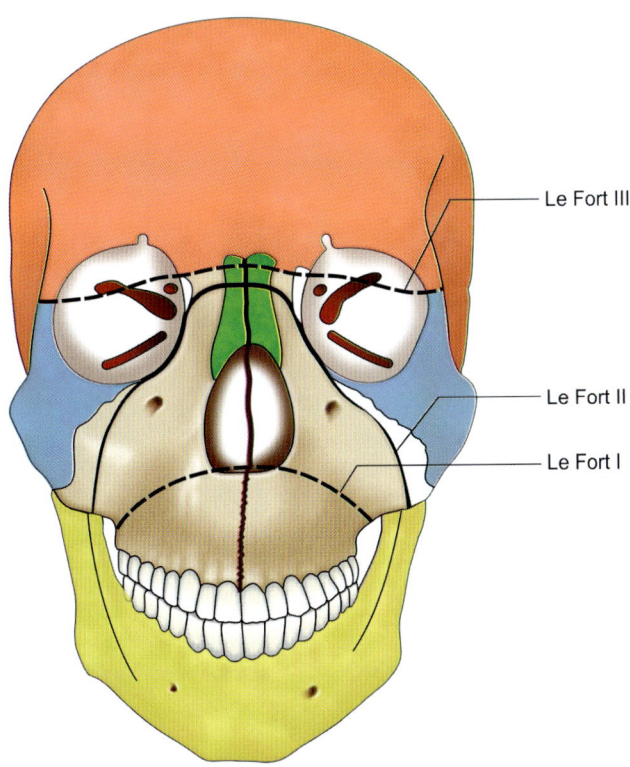

**Fig. 10.4:** Common fractures of maxillae and other bones

B. Bilateral maxillary fractures are classified into following three types:

    *a. Le Fort I (Guerin's fracture)*

      It is a horizontal fracture along the floor of nose and below the zygomatic bone.

    *b. Le Fort II*

      In this fracture line passes through orbits then runs medial to and below the zygomatic bones towards the alveolar margins.

    *c. Le Fort III*

      In this, the fracture line runs through nasal bones and orbits above the zygomatic bone. This fracture is also called craniofacial disjunction as the face separates from cranium.

# 11

# Parietal Bones

## TERMINOLOGY

The word parietal is derived from Latin word 'paries' which means 'wall', because two parietal bones form large part of walls of calvaria.

## SIDE DETERMINATION

1. Keep the bone by the side of your own cranial vault in such a way that outer surface is convex and inner surface is concave.

2. Inferior (squamosal) border is concave.

3. Anteroinferior angle is prominent and has got a vascular and narrow groove on its inner aspect.

4. The posteroinferior angle has got a shallow and wide groove for sigmoid sinus on its inner aspect.

## FEATURES AND ATTACHMENTS

### I. Surfaces

It has two surfaces, external and internal.

*A. External surface* **(Fig. 11.1)**

   1. It is relatively smooth.

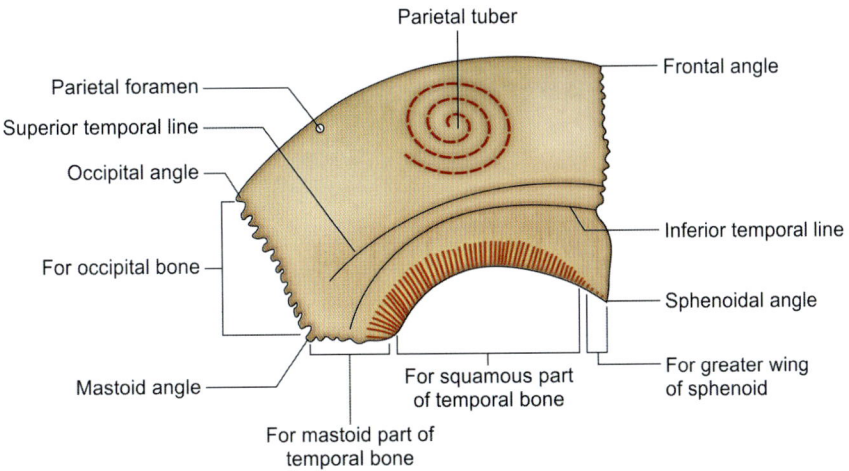

**Fig. 11.1:** Right parietal bone: External surface

2. Most prominent part of this surface is called *parietal tuberosity* or *eminence*.

3. There are two curved lines running anteroposteriorly. These are called *superior and inferior temporal lines*. Superior temporal line gives attachment to *tempral fascia* while area below inferior temporal line gives attachment to *temporalis muscle*.

4. Area above the superior temporal line is covered by *galea aponeurotica*.

5. A foramen may be present near the posterior part of sagittal border. This is called *parietal foramen*. It transmits *emissary vein*.

B. *Internal surface* (Fig. 11.2)

1. It is concave and exhibits elevations and depressions for cerebral sulci and gyri respectively.

2. Near the sagittal border there is a longitudinal half groove (to be completed with that of opposite side) for *superior sagittal sinus*. The margins of groove provide attachment to *falx cerebri*.

3. Grooves for the branches of *middle meningeal vessels* are present at the anteroinferior angle and at the middle of the lower border of the bone.

4. Adjacent to groove for superior sagittal sinus there are deep irregular pits (*granular foveolae*) produced by *arachnoid granulations*.

5. The bone is grooved near the postero-inferior angle by *sigmoid sinus*.

## II. Borders

It has four borders, superior, inferior, anterior and posterior.

A. *Superior border*

1. This is also called sagittal border.

2. It articulates with the similar border of opposite side to form sagittal suture.

B. *Inferior border*

1. This is also called squamosal border.

2. It articulates with following three bones from anterior to posterior:
   i. Greater wing of sphenoid.
   ii. Squamous part of temporal.
   iii. Mastoid portion of temporal.

C. *Anterior border*

1. This is also called frontal border.

2. It articulates with the frontal bone to form *coronal suture*.

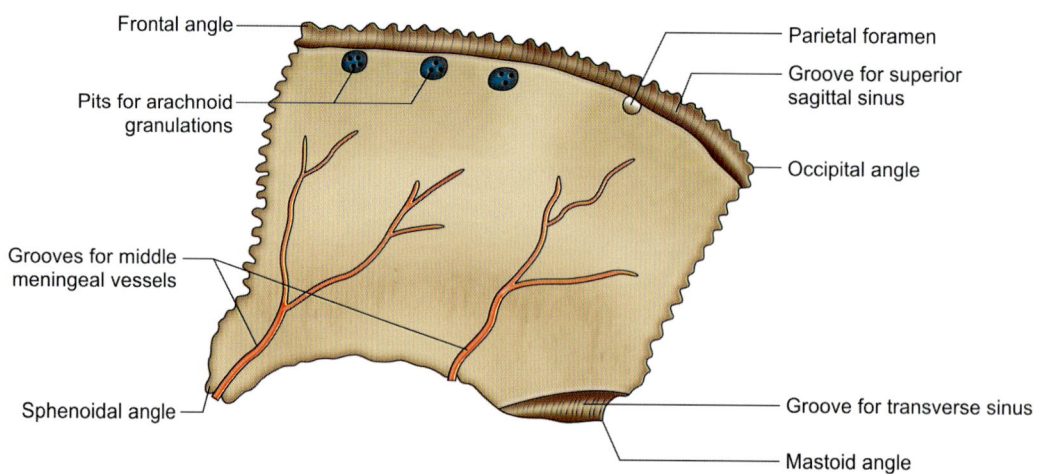

**Fig. 11.2:** Right parietal bone: Internal surface

## D. Posterior border

1. This is also called occipital border.
2. It articulates with the squamous part of occipital bone to form *lambdoid suture*.

## III. Angles

Parietal bone has four angles (frontal, sphenoidal, occipital and mastoid).

### A. Frontal angle

1. This is also called anterosuperior angle.
2. It corresponds to *bregma*, i.e. the junction of coronal and sagittal sutures.

### B. Sphenoidal angle

1. This is also called anteroinferior angle.
2. It correspsonds to *pterion*, i.e. a small area enclosing four bones (frontal, temporal, parietal and greater wing of sphenoid).

### C. Occipital angle

1. This is also called posterosuperior angle.
2. It corresponds to *lambda*, i.e. junction of sagittal and lambdoid sutures.

### D. Mastoid angle

1. This is also called posteroinferior angle.
2. It corresponds to *asterion*, i.e. small area enclosing three bones, parietal, temporal and occipital.

## OSSIFICATION

1. Parietal bones ossify in membrane.
2. Each ossifies from two centres which appear at parietal tuberosity at about 7th week of intrauterine life.
3. The centres soon fuse with each other and then the ossification spreads radially.
4. Angles are the parts last to be ossified explaining the existence of a fontanelle at each angle before the ossification is completed.

## AGE CHANGES

1. **At birth**
   Temporal lines are present at quite a lower level.
2. **Adult**
   A higher and permanent positions of temporal lines are reached only after the eruption of permanent molar teeth.

## APPLIED ANATOMY

1. Occasionally the parietal bone is divided into upper and lower parts by an anteroposterior suture. The condition may be confused with fracture radiologically. The latter can be ruled out easily because the anomalous parietal suture is usually bilateral.

2. Parietal bones are loosely attached to the adjacent bones at sutures during intrauterine period allowing moulding (change in shape of calvaria) at the time of child birth. Calvaria returns to normal shape within few days after birth.

3. Parietal bones undergo remodelling to allow enlargement of calvaria during childhood. This is only possible because of their loose attachments to the adjacent bones.

4. *Granular foveolae* are more numerous and marked in aged parietal bones. This fact is of great medicolegal importance.

5. Regenerating capacity of the parietal bone is negligible due to lack of cambium layer in periosteum.

6. In neonates the parietal bone is pliable and soft and, therefore, a *depressed fracture (pond fracture)* is like a dimple. In adults such fractures are produced by direct blows and always show an irregular line of fracture at the periphery of depressed area (Fig. 11.3). The depression of the inner table forms the

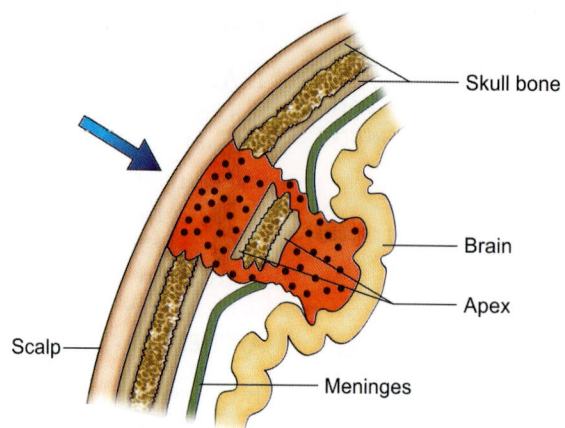

Skull bone

Brain

Apex

Scalp

Meninges

**Fig. 11.3:** A depressed fracture of parietal bone in adult

lowest limit of the depressed area also known as apex.

7. A crack in the inner table of parietal bone may damage a large diploeic vein and produce small *epidural haematoma*.

8. Almost invariably all fractures of the parietal bone in children are associated with rupture of dura mater.

9. In adult the parietal bone shows a fissured or linear fracture if the force is transmitted to this bone from frontal or occipital blows.

# 12

# Frontal Bone

## TERMINOLOGY

The term 'frontal' is derived from Latin word 'frons' which means 'brow' or 'forehead'.

## LOCATION

Frontal bone forms the forehead, greater part of the roof of each orbit and most of the floor of anterior cranial fossa.

## FEATURES AND ATTACHMENTS

Frontal bone has got a main part (frontal squama) and orbital parts.

### I. Frontal squama (main part)

It has got an external surface, right and left temporal surfaces, an internal surface, a nasal part and a margin (parietal or posterior).

### A. Surfaces

*a. External surface* (Figs 12.1 and 12.2)

   i. *Supra-orbital margins.*
   1. These are lower limits of external surface on each side.
   2. They form upper borders of the orbital openings.
   ii. *Supra-orbital notch or foramen*
   1. The junction of lateral two-thirds of supra-orbital margin (sharp) with the medial one-third (rounded) is marked by supra-orbital notch (some times foramen).
   2. This is meant for the passage of *supra-orbital nerve, supra-orbital artery* and *a communicating vein* between angular and superior ophthalmic veins.
   iii. *Superciliary arch*
   This is an arched prominence just above the supra-orbital margin.
   iv. *Glabella*
   It is the median prominence between superciliary arches.
   v. *Frontal eminence*
   1. On each side, about 3 cm above the supra-orbital margin, there is an elevated area called frontal eminence or tuberosity.
   2. It is usually more marked in female.
   vi. *Metopic suture*
   Frontal bone is bilateral in origin and the junction of the two halves is called frontal or metopic suture. Its remains can be seen even in adult in the reigon of glabella.
   vii. *Zygomatic process*
   1. Supra-orbital margin extends laterally on each side into a zygomatic process.
   2. Zygomatic process articulates with frontal process of zygomatic bone.

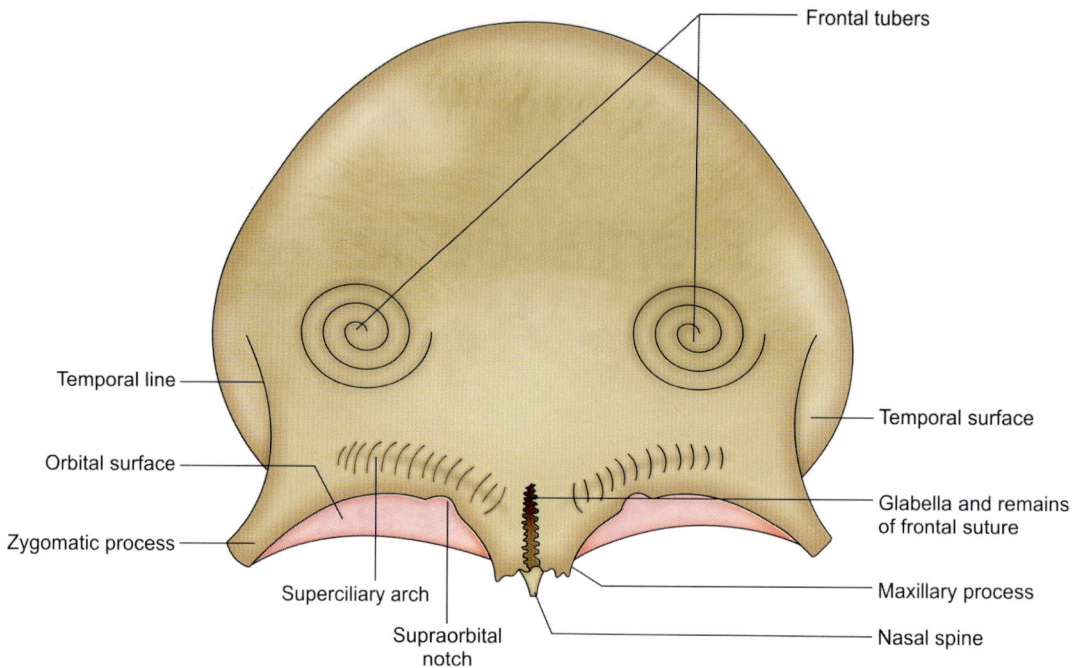

Frontal tubers

Temporal line

Orbital surface

Zygomatic process

Superciliary arch

Supraorbital notch

Temporal surface

Glabella and remains of frontal suture

Maxillary process

Nasal spine

**Fig. 12.1:** Frontal bone: Anterior aspect

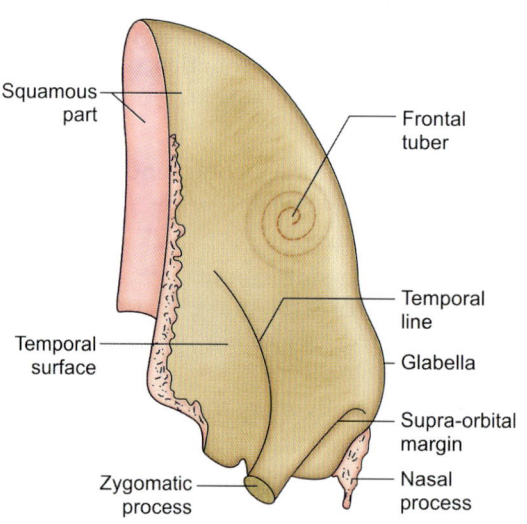

Squamous part

Frontal tuber

Temporal line

Glabella

Temporal surface

Supra-orbital margin

Zygomatic process

Nasal process

**Fig. 12.2:** Frontal bone: Right lateral aspect

viii. A line curves upwards and backwards from the zyomatic process. The line soon divides into two lines called *superior and inferior temporal lines.*

### b. Temporal surfaces

1. An area on each side below and behind the temporal lines is called temporal surface.

2. It contributes to the anterior part of *temporal fossa* on the lateral aspect of skull (norma lateralis).

3. Superior temporal line gives attachment to *temporal fascia.*

4. Inferior temporal line and temporal surface of frontal bone give origin to *temporalis muscle.*

### c. Internal surface (Fig. 12.3)

i. This surface shows depressions and elevations for cerebral gyri and sulci respectively.

ii. *Sagittal sulcus*

1. It is a midline sulcus in the upper part of internal surface.

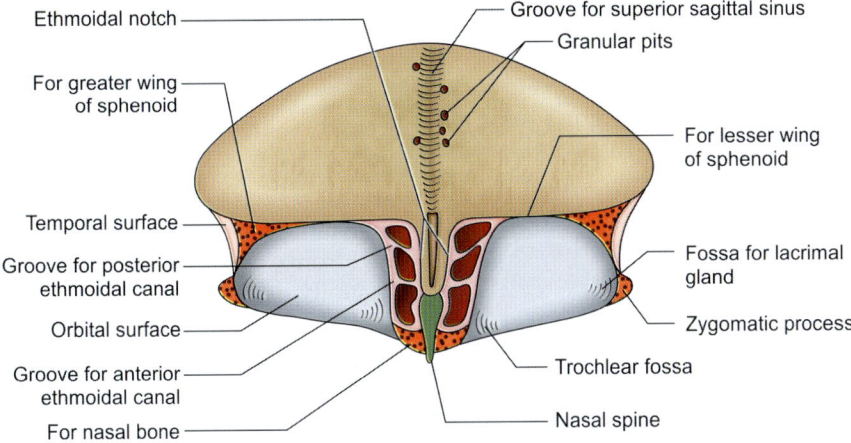

Ethmoidal notch
For greater wing of sphenoid
Temporal surface
Groove for posterior ethmoidal canal
Orbital surface
Groove for anterior ethmoidal canal
For nasal bone

Groove for superior sagittal sinus
Granular pits
For lesser wing of sphenoid
Fossa for lacrimal gland
Zygomatic process
Trochlear fossa
Nasal spine

**Fig. 12.3:** Frontal bone: Inferior aspect

2. Its margins provide attachments to *falx cerebri.*
3. Sulcus itself lodges *superior sagittal sinus.*

iii. *Frontal crest*
1. Margins of sagittal sulcus meet in the midline in the lower part and continue as frontal crest.
2. This also gives attachment to *falx cerebri.*

iv. A notch below the frontal crest is converted into *foramen caecum* by articulation with ethmoid bone. An *emissary vein* passing through it connects the vein of nose with superior sagittal sinus.

v. Several depressions (*granular foveolae*) on each side of sagittal sulcus are produced by *arachnoid granulations.*

### B. Nasal part
1. It is a downward projection of frontal bone between two supra-orbital margins.
2. Its lower serrated part is known as *nasal notch.*
3. Each half of the nasal notch articulates with the following three bones from anterior to posterior:

i. *Nasal bone.*
ii. *Frontal process of maxilla.*
iii. *Lacrimal bone.*

4. *Nasal spine* is a midline downward continuation of the nasal part.
5. On each side of nasal spine there is a grooved area which froms the roof of nasal cavity.
6. Nasal spine itself articulates with crest of the nasal bone anteriorly and perpendicular plate of ethmoid posteriorly.

### C. Posterior margin
1. This is also called parietal margin because its major part articulates with *parietal bones.*
2. The lower part of this margin is triangular and rough for articulation with *greater wing of sphenoid.*

### II. Orbital parts
Orbital parts consist of two triangular laminae (*orbital plates*) separated by a gap called *ethmoidal notch.*

### A. Orbital plate
It possesses two surfaces, orbital and internal.

### a. Orbital surface

1. It faces downwards.
2. It forms *roof of the orbit*.
3. Its anterolateral part has got a *fossa for the lacrimal gland*.
4. Its anteromedial part (*trochlear fovea*) provides attachment to *fibrocartilaginous pulley* for tendon of superior oblique muscle.

### b. Internal surface (Fig. 12.4)

1. It faces upwards.
2. It contributes to anterior cranial fossa.
3. It has impressions for gyri of frontal lobe of cerebral hemisphere.
4. It has grooves for meningeal vessels.

### B. Ethmoidal notch (Figs 12.3 and 12.4)

1. It is 'U' shaped gap occupied by *cribriform plate of ethmoid*.
2. Under surfaces of its lateral margins possess several incomplete air cells which complete the ethmiodal air cells when ethmoid bone is in position.
3. Two grooves on the under surface of each margin are converted into *anterior and posterior ethmoidal canals* by similar grooves on the superior surface of ethmoidal labyrinth. These canals are meant for passages of *anterior and posterior ethmoidal nerves and vessels*.

4. The under surface of the anterior margin of the notch possesses openings for frontal sinuses (one on each side of the nasal spine).

### III. Frontal sinus

Each frontal sinus is an irregular cavity of variable size. It is situated between outer and inner tables of frontal bone. They are separated from each other by a bony septum which is usually deviated to one side.

### OSSIFICATION

1. Frontal bone ossifies in membrane.
2. Two primary centres appear, one for each half of frontal bone, in the region of frontal tuberosity.
3. Primary centres appear during 8th week of intrauterine life.
4. Ossification extends upwards to form frontal squama, backwards to form orbital part and downwards to form nasal part.
5. At birth frontal bone is made up of two halves separated by *frontal* or *metopic suture* (Fig. 12.5).
6. Union between two parts begins at 2nd year and completes at 8th year.

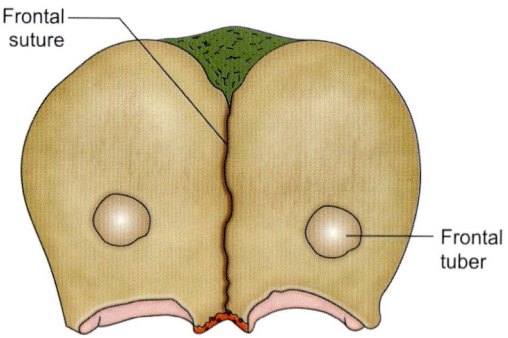

Fig. 12.5: Frontal bone at birth

### APPLIED ANATOMY

1. Frontal squama is soft and pliable in neonates which can withstand considerable amount of compression and moulding, a fact clinically important during child birth.

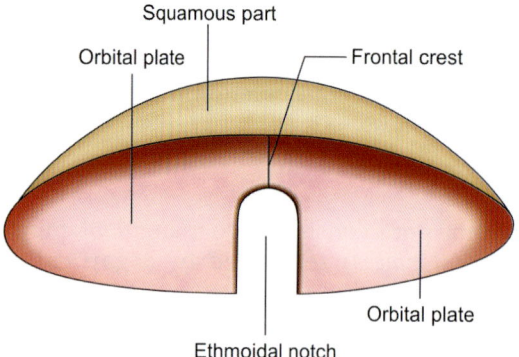

**Fig. 12.4:** Frontal bone: Superior aspect (diagrammatic)

2. Frontal squama is prone to depressed or fissured fractures. In neonates and infants, the depressed fracture is often like a dimple in the bone. In adults a depressed fracture is always associated with irregular line of fracture.
3. A severe impact at the root of the nose leads to fractures of frontal sinus walls (Fig. 12.6). If the fracture involves inner table forming the posterior wall of frontal sinus, then the air may enter into the cranial cavity (*aerocele*) causing meningitis and brain abscess.
4. *Fracture of orbital plate of frontal bone* causes haemorrhages into the orbit. The haemorrhage aquires a triangular shape under the conjunctiva whose apex is towards the corneoscleral junction and base towards the orbital margin (Fig. 12.7).

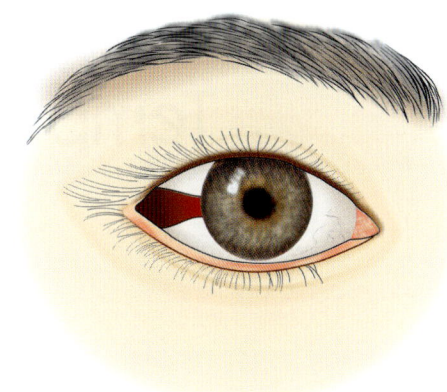

**Fig. 12.7:** A triangular haemorrhagic appearance whose exact peripheral limit is not visible (orbital plate fracture)

5. A crack in the inner table of frontal squama may damage a large diploeic vein and produce small *epidural haematoma*.
6. Almost invariably the fractures of frontal squama in children are associated with rupture of dura mater.
7. A gap in frontal squama will not be regenerating and has to be filled with tantalum or titanium, a procedure called *cranial prosthesis.*

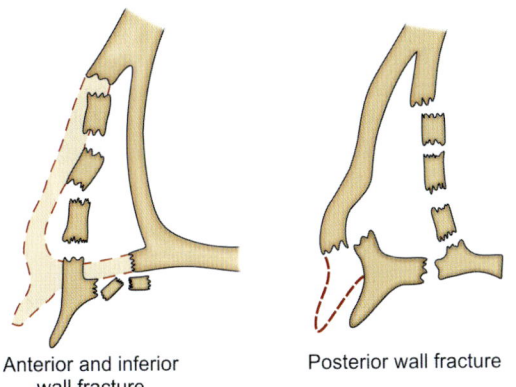

Anterior and inferior wall fracture — Posterior wall fracture

**Fig. 12.6:** Fracture of frontal sinus walls

# CHAPTER

# 13

# Temporal Bones

## TERMINOLOGY

Temporal bone is so named because of its contribution to temporal region.

## SIDE DETERMINATION

I. To distinguish superior and inferior, following features are to be noted:
   1. Thin plate like squamous part is directed upwards and lies in para-sagittal plane.
   2. Styloid and mastoid processes occupy the lower part of the bone and are directed downwards.

II. To distinguish external and internal aspects, one should consider following features:
   1. The outer surface of squamous part is very smooth.
   2. Zygomatic process is present on the external aspect of bone.
   3. External acoustic meatus (present below the posterior part of zygomatic process) opens externally.
   4. Apex of petrous temporal is directed medially and a little forwards.

III. To distinguish anterior from posterior, following criteria should be taken into account:

1. Zygomatic process is directed forwards.
2. Mandibular fossa and external acoustic meatus are present below the posterior part of zygomatic process. Relatively, mandibular fossa is anterior to external acoustic meatus.

## FEATURES AND ATTACHMENTS

Morphologically temporal bone is divided into four parts.

1. *Squamous part.*
2. *Petromastoid part.*
3. *Tympanic part.*
4. *Styloid process.*

For descriptive purpose, the petromastoid part is further subdivided into mastoid part and petrous part.

### I. SQUAMOUS PART

It is thin and plate like and occupies anterior and superior part of temporal bone. It has two surfaces (temporal and cerebral) and two borders (superior and anteroinferior).

### A. Surfaces

*a. Temporal surface* (Fig. 13.1)
   1. It is outer surface.
   2. It is smooth and slightly convex.

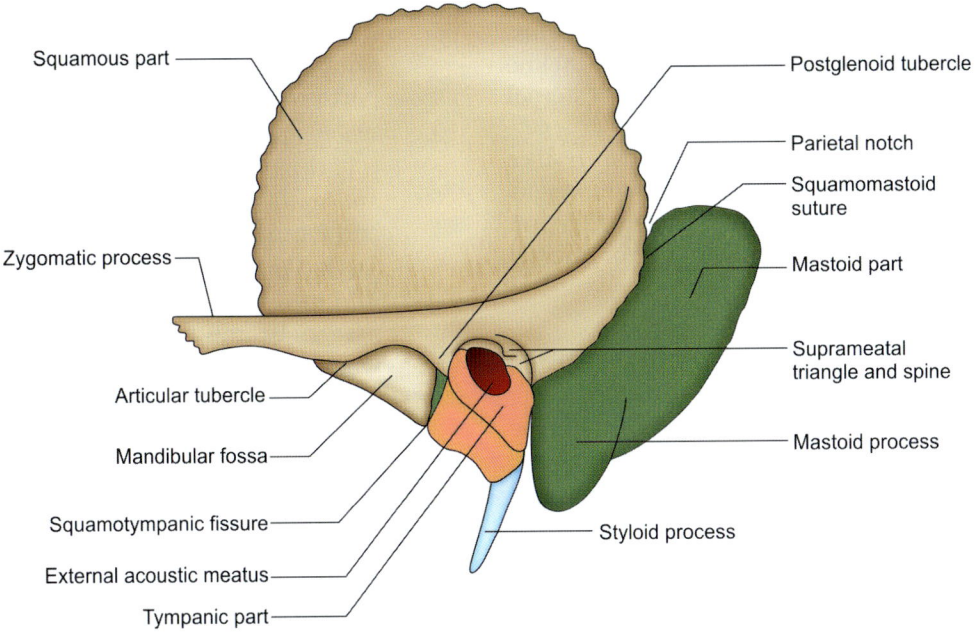

**Fig. 13.1:** Left temporal bone: External aspect

3. It contributes to the temporal fossa meant for the origin of *temporalis muscle.*

4. *Middle temporal artery* grooves the surface, just above the external acoustic meatus.

5. *Supramastoid crest* runs backwards and upwards across its posterior part. Temporal fascia is attached to this crest.

6. *Squamomastoid suture* marks the junction between squamous and mastoid parts. It is situated 1.5 cm. below the supramastoid crest.

7. *Macewen's triangle (suprameatal triangle)* (Fig. 13.2)

   i. It is a triangular depression postero-superior to external acoustic meatus.

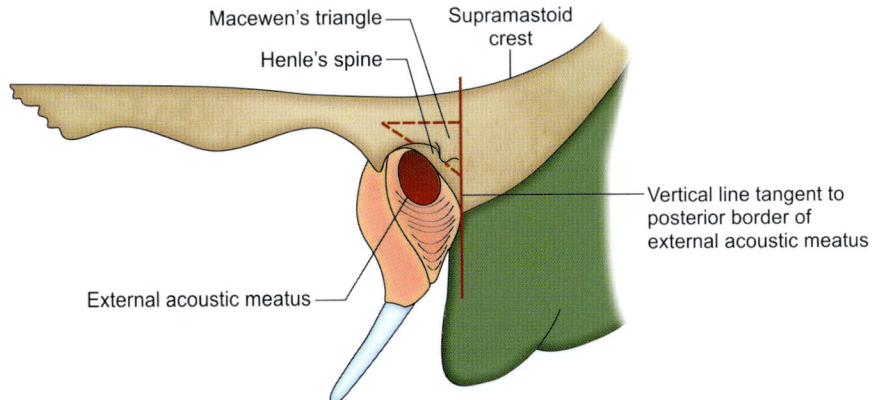

**Fig. 13.2:** Macewen's triangle of left side

ii. It is bounded by posterosuperior margin of external acoustic meatus, supramastoid crest and a vertical line tangent to posterior border of external acoustic meatus.

iii. *Spine of Henle* is sharp, spur like projection in the suprameatal triangle.

iv. Mastoid antrum is situated 12.5 mm deep to the surface of suprameatal triangle in adult.

8. *Zygomatic process*

  i. It is a forward projection from the lower part of temporal surface.

  ii. Its anterior end articulates with the temporal process of zygomatic bone to complete the zygomatic arch or zygoma.

  iii. Anterior part of zygomatic process has two surfaces (lateral and medial) and two borders (superior and inferior). *Masseter* originates from its medial surface and inferior border. *Temporal fascia* is attached to its superior border. Its lateral surface is subcutaneous.

  iv. Its posterior part is triangular having superior and inferior surfaces.

  v. Inferior surface of the posterior part of zygomatic process is bounded by two roots (anterior and posterior) which converge at the *tubercle of the root of zygoma*. Lateral *ligament of temporomandibular joint* is attached to this tubercle.

  vi. Anterior root extends medially from tubercle of the root of zygoma and is also called *articular tubercle*.

9. *Mandibular fossa*

  i. It is situated behind the articular tubercle.

  ii. Only anterior part of mandibular fossa is articular and contributed by squamous part of temporal bone.

  iii. Articular tubercle and anterior part of mandibular fossa is related to the superior surface of *articular disc* of temporomandibular joint.

  iv. Posterior part of mandibular fossa is non-articular and contributed by tympanic part of temporal bone. This part is related to the *parotid gland*.

10. *Squamotympanic fissure*

  i. It is situated in the mandibular fossa and marks the junction of squamous and tympanic parts of temporal bone.

  ii. Medial part of this fissure is divided into *petrosquamous and petrotympanic fissures* by the projection of *tegmen tympani* of petrous part of temporal bone.

  iii. Three structures pass through petro-tympanic fissure, i.e. *chorda tympani nerve, anterior tympanic artery* and *anterior ligament of malleus*.

**Note:** *To remember the structures passing through petrotympanic fissure think of a 'CAT' in which C—Chorda tympani nerve, A—Anterior ligament of malleus and T—Tympanic artery.*

  iv. Petrotympanic fissure leads into middle ear.

b. *Cerebral surface*

  1. It is inner surface.

  2. It is grooved by *middle meningeal vessels*.

  3. It has impressions for sulci and gyri of the temporal lobe of cerebrum.

## B. Borders

a. *Superior border*

It articulates with parietal bone.

b. *Anteroinferior border*

It articulates with greater wing of sphenoid bone.

## II. MASTOID PART

It forms the posterior part of the temporal bone. It consists of two surfaces (outer and inner), two borders (superior and posterior) and a downward projecting part called mastoid process.

## A. Surfaces

### a. Outer surface

1. *Auricularis posterior* and *occipital belly of occipitofrontalis* are attached to this surface.
2. *Mastoid foramen* is an infrequent opening near the posterior border. When present this foramen transmits an *emissary vein* from sigmoid sinus and a *branch from occipital artery*.

### b. Inner surface

1. *Sigmoid sulcus* is a deep groove on the inner surface. It is meant for *sigmoid sinus*.
2. *Mastoid foramen* opens in the upper part of sigmoid sulcus.

## B. Borders

### a. Superior border

It articulates with the occipital bone at *occipitomastoid suture*.

### b. Posterior border

It articulates with the occipital bone at *occipitomastoid suture*.

## C. Mastoid process

It possesses a lateral and a medial surface.

### a. Lateral surface

It gives insertions to following three muscles from above downwards:

1. *Sternomastoid*.
2. *Splenius capitis*.
3. *Longissimus capitis*.

### b. Medial surface

1. It is marked by a deep groove called *mastoid notch*, from which originates the *posterior belly of digastric*.
2. *Occipital groove* is observed medial to mastoid notch. This groove lodges the *occipital artery*.

## III. PETROUS PART

Petrous is a Latin word which means strong or rock like. It is strong part of temporal bone and protects internal ear within it. Petrous part is comprised of a base, an apex, three surfaces (anterior, posterior and inferior) and three borders (superior, anterior and posterior).

### A. Base

1. It is directed laterally.
2. It fuses with squamous part at petrosquamosal suture which disappears soon after birth.
3. Base also fuses with mastoid part.
4. Base is separated from the squamous and mastoid parts by an air filled space called *mastoid antrum*.

### B. Apex

1. It projects medially and slightly forwards.
2. It is situated between greater wing of sphenoid and basilar part of occipital bone.
3. It forms posterolateral boundary of foramen lacerum.
4. It possesses anterior orifice of carotid canal.

### C. Surfaces

#### a. Anterior surface (Fig. 13.3)

1. It contributes to middle cranial fossa.
2. This surface shows following features if one goes from apex to base:
   i. *Trigeminal impression*: It is a depression for trigeminal ganglion adjacent to apex.
   ii. *Roof of internal acoustic meatus*: It is another depressed area behind the ridge.
   iii. *Arcuate eminence*: It is a prominent elevation produced by superior semicircular canal. Its posterior sloping lies over lateral and posterior semicircular canals.

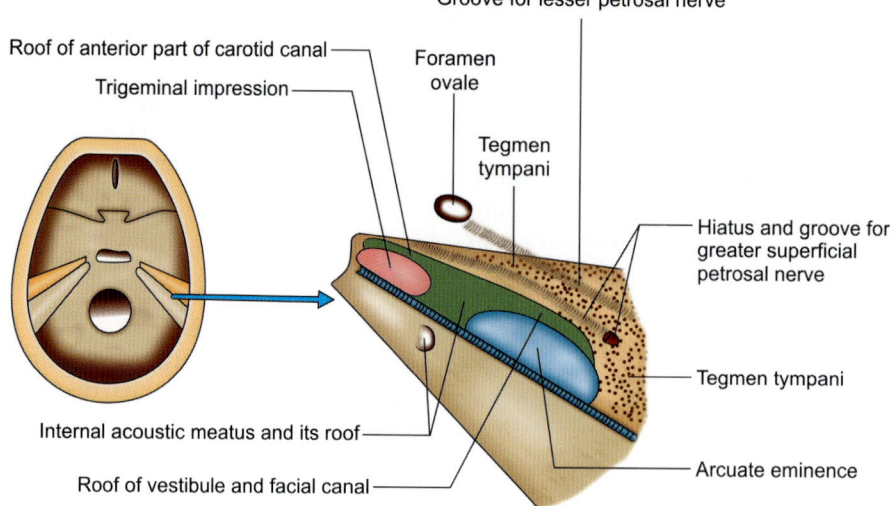

Groove for lesser petrosal nerve

Roof of anterior part of carotid canal

Foramen ovale

Trigeminal impression

Tegmen tympani

Hiatus and groove for greater superficial petrosal nerve

Tegmen tympani

Internal acoustic meatus and its roof

Arcuate eminence

Roof of vestibule and facial canal

**Fig. 13.3:** Anterior surface of petrous part of right temporal bone

3. Area anterolateral to trigeminal impression forms the roof of *anterior part of carotid canal.*

4. Area anterolateral to arcuate eminence forms the roof of vestibule and beginning of *facial canal.*

5. Thin plate of bone between squamous part (cerebral surface) of temporal bone and features described above is called *tegmen tympani.* It forms roof of mastoid antrum, middle ear and canal for tensor tympani from posterior to anterior. Tegmen tympani projects downwards to form lateral walls of canal for tensor tympani and bony Eustachian tube and appears in the squamotympanic fissure.

6. A hiatus (opening) lateral to arcuate eminence leads into a *groove for greater superficial petrosal nerve* which runs towards the foramen lacerum on the tegmen tympani.

7. Lateral to groove for greater superficial petrosal nerve is present a *groove for lesser petrosal nerve* which runs towards the foramen ovale.

*b. Posterior surface* (Fig. 13.4)

1. It contributes to posterior cranial fossa.

2. *Internal acoustic meatus* is present in the centre of this surface. It transmits *facial and vestibulocochlear nerves* and *labyrinthine vessels.* It is about 1 cm in length.

3. *Fundus* of internal acoustic meatus is a plate of bone at its lateral end. This plate is divided into upper and lower areas by a transverse ridge called *crista falciformis.* The upper area is further divided into anterior and posterior areas by a vertical crest called *Bill's bar.* Anterior area shows *facial canal* for facial nerve. Posterior area is called *superior vestibular* area which presents number of small openings for the nerve fibres supplying utricle and superior and lateral semicircular ducts (Fig. 13.5).

Below the transverse crest, anteriorly is the *cochlear area* (which possesses number of foramina called *tractus spiralis foraminosus*) and posteriorly is the *inferior vestibular* area. Fibres of cochlear nerve

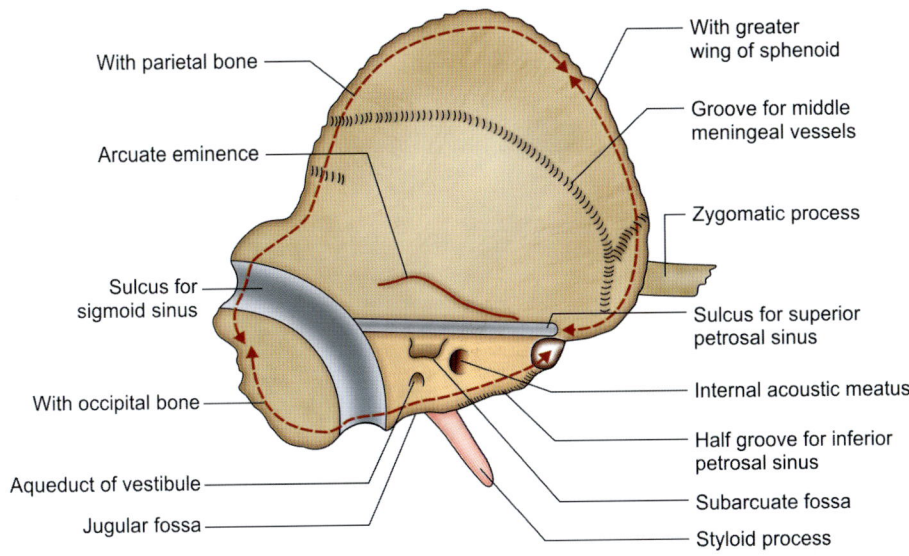

**Fig. 13.4:** Left temporal bone: Internal aspect

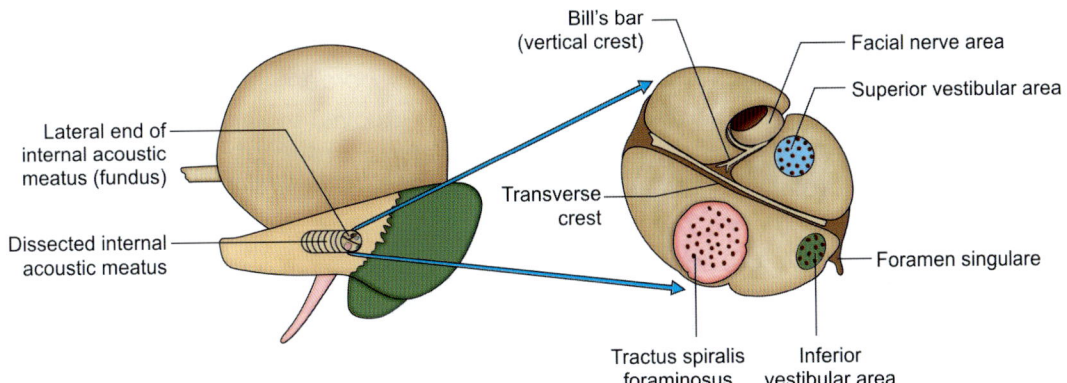

**Fig. 13.5:** Fundus of right internal acoustic meatus

enter the cochlear area while nerve fibres supplying the saccule enter the inferior vestibular area. Below and behind the inferior vestibular area is *foramen singulare* for the passage of nerve to posterior semicircular duct.

4. A slit behind the internal acoustic meatus leads into *aqueduct of vestibule* which contains saccus and ductus endolymphaticus along with small artery and vein.

5. An irregular depression called *subarcuate fossa* is located above and between the openings of internal acoustic meatus and aqueduct of vestibule. It lodges a process of dura mater.

*c. Inferior surface* (Fig. 13.6)

1. It is rough and triangular.

2. It is divided into four areas from apex to base.

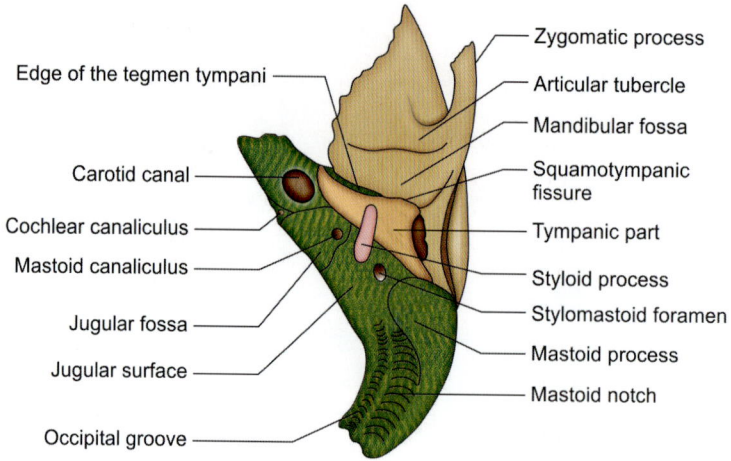

**Fig. 13.6:** Left temporal bone: Inferior aspect

i. *Quadrilateral area* near the apex provides attachment to *levator palati muscle.*

ii. *Carotid canal* (lower opening) is present behind the quadrilateral area. It transmits *internal carotid artery* along with its *sympathetic* and *venous plexuses.*

iii. *Jugular fossa* is a depression behind the carotid canal. It lodges *superior bulb of internal jugular vein.*

iv. *Jugular surface* is a quadrilateral area behind the jugular fossa. It articulates with jugular process of occipital bone.

3. A triangular depression in front of the medial part of the jugular fossa lodges the *inferior ganglion of glossopharyngeal nerve.* The apex of this triangular depression is marked by an opening leading into *cochlear canaliculus* which is traversed by:

    i. *Perilymphatic duct*

    ii. *Prolongation of dura mater*

    iii. A *vein* from cochlea which drains into internal jugular vein.

4. The *canaliculus for tympanic nerve* (a branch of glossopharyngeal nerve) is situated on the bony ridge between carotid canal and jugular fossa.

5. The *mastoid canaliculus* is present in the lateral wall of jugular fossa. It transmits the *auricular branch of vagus.*

### D. Borders

#### a. Superior border

1. It is grooved by *superior petrosal sinus.*
2. Margins of the groove provide attachment to *tentorium cerebelli.*

#### b. Anterior border

1. It is divided into medial and lateral parts.
2. Medial part articulates with greater wing of sphenoid.
3. Lateral part joins the squamous part at *petrosquamosal suture* which disappears soon after birth.

#### c. Posterior border

1. It can be divided into medial and lateral parts.
2. Medial part has got a sulcus which with similar sulcus on the occipital bone forms a *groove for inferior petrosal sinus.*
3. Lateral part is occupied by larger *jugular fossa* laterally and smaller *glossopharyngeal notch* medially. Lateral part forms *anterior boundary of jugular foramen* whose posterior boundary is formed by jugular notch of occipital bone.

## IV. TYMPANIC PART

It is curved bony plate situated below the squamous part and in front of mastoid part of temporal bone. It joins the squamous part at *squamotympanic fissure* and mastoid part at *tympanomastoid fissure*. Auricular branch of vagus emerges through the tympanomastoid fissure. Tympanic part has two surfaces (anterior and posterior) and three borders (lateral, upper and lower).

### A. Surfaces

#### a. Anterior surface

1. It forms the posterior nonarticular part of the *mandibular fossa*.
2. It is related to the *parotid gland*.

#### b. Posterior surface

1. It forms the anterior wall, floor and the lower part of the posterior wall of the *external acoustic meatus*.
2. Its medial end is marked by a groove called *tympanic sulcus*. This sulcus provides attachment to the circumference of the *tympanic membrane*.

### B. Borders

#### a. Lateral border

1. It is free.
2. It continues with cartilaginous part of external acoustic meatus.

#### b. Upper border

1. Laterally it fuses with the *postglenoid tubercle*.
2. Medially it forms posterior boundary of *petrotympanic fissure*.

#### c. Lower border

1. Medially it extends upto carotid canal.
2. Laterally it splits to form the veginal process which encloses the root of styloid process.

## V. STYLOID PROCESS

1. Styloid process is divisible into two parts: Proximal and Distal.

#### a. *Proximal or tympanohyal part*

It is surrounded by a bony sheath derived from lower border of tympanic part of temporal bone.

#### b. *Distal or stylohyal part*

It is visible lower part. It is this part which is described below.

2. Styloid process is a conical projection directed downwards, forwards and slightly medially.
3. It provides attachments to five structures (3 muscles and 2 ligaments):
    i. Medially: *Stylopharyngeus muscle.*
    ii. Anteriorly: *Styloglossus muscle.*
    iii. Posteriorly: *Stylohyoid muscle.*
    iv. Laterally: *Stylomandibular ligament.*
    v. At the tip: *Stylohyoid ligament.*
4. Some important relations are as follows:
    i. It is interposed between two important structures, the *parotid gland* (laterally) and *internal jugular vein* (medially).
    ii. *External carotid* artery crosses the tip of styloid process superficially .
    iii. *Facial nerve* crosses the base of styloid process laterally.
5. *Stylomastoid foramen* is situated behind its base (between it and the mastoid process). Following structures pass through this foramen:
    i. *Facial nerve.*
    ii. *Stylomastoid artery.*

## SPACES AND CANALS

## I. External acoustic meatus (Fig. 13.7)

1. Bony part of external acoustic meatus is about 16 mm long. This contribution is about 2/3rd of the total length (24 mm).
2. It is directed medially, downwards and slightly forwards.
3. Tympanic part of the temporal bone contributes to its anterior wall, floor and lower part of the posterior wall.
4. Squamous part of the temporal bone forms its roof and upper part of posterior wall.

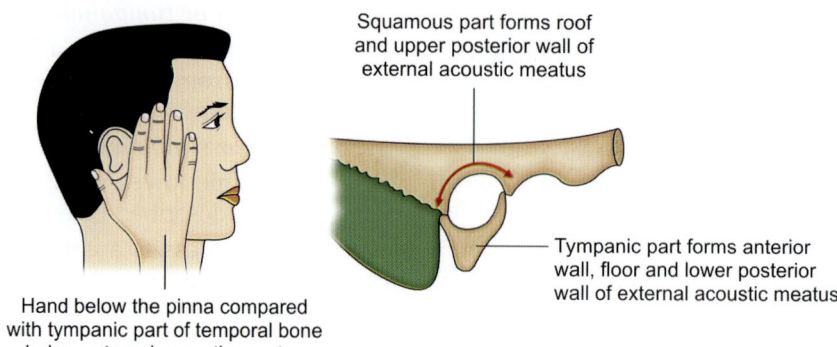

Squamous part forms roof and upper posterior wall of external acoustic meatus

Tympanic part forms anterior wall, floor and lower posterior wall of external acoustic meatus

Hand below the pinna compared with tympanic part of temporal bone below external acoustic meatus

**Fig. 13.7:** Bony contributions to external acoustic meatus: Right lateral view

## II. Middle ear space (tympanic cavity)

### A. Parts

Tympanic cavity consists of three parts:

a. *Tympanic cavity proper (mesotympanum):* Opposite the tympanic membrane.

b. *Epitympanic recess (epitympanum):* Above the level of the tympanic membrane.

c. *Hypotympanum:* Below the level of the tympanic membrane.

### B. Measurements

1. Vertical diameter – 15 mm.

2. Anteroposterior diameter – 15 mm.

3. Transverse diameters:

   i. Upper part – 6 mm.

   ii. Lower part – 4 mm.

   iii. Opposite the centre of tympanic membrane – 2 mm.

### C. Boundaries

#### a. Roof

It is formed by *tegmen tympani* which separates the middle ear from middle cranial fossa.

#### b. Floor

It is formed by thin plate of bone which separates the cavity from *superior bulb of internal jugular vein.*

### c. Lateral wall (Fig. 13.8)

1. It is formed mainly by *tympanic membrane.*

2. Close to circumference for tympanic membrane there are three small apertures:

   i. *Petrotympanic fissure*: It is located anteriorly.

   ii. *Anterior canaliculus for chorda tympani*: It is located at the medial end of petrotympanic fissure.

   iii. *Posterior canaliculus for chorda tympani*: It is located posteriorly.

### d. Medial wall (Fig. 13.9)

1. It is the lateral wall of internal ear.

2. It has a rounded elevation called *promontory* produced by the basal turn of cochlea.

3. Promontory is grooved by the nerves of *tympanic plexus.*

4. A depression behind the promontory, the *sinus tympani*, indicates the position of the *ampulla of the posterior semicircular canal.*

5. *Fenestra vestibuli* is a reniform opening posterosuperior to the promontory. It connects the tympanic cavity to the vestibule of internal ear.

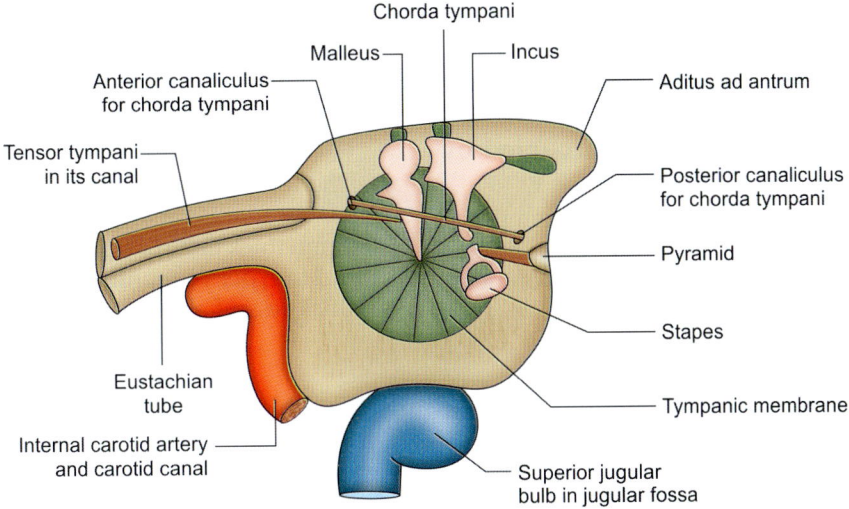

**Fig. 13.8:** Lateral wall of middle ear of right side

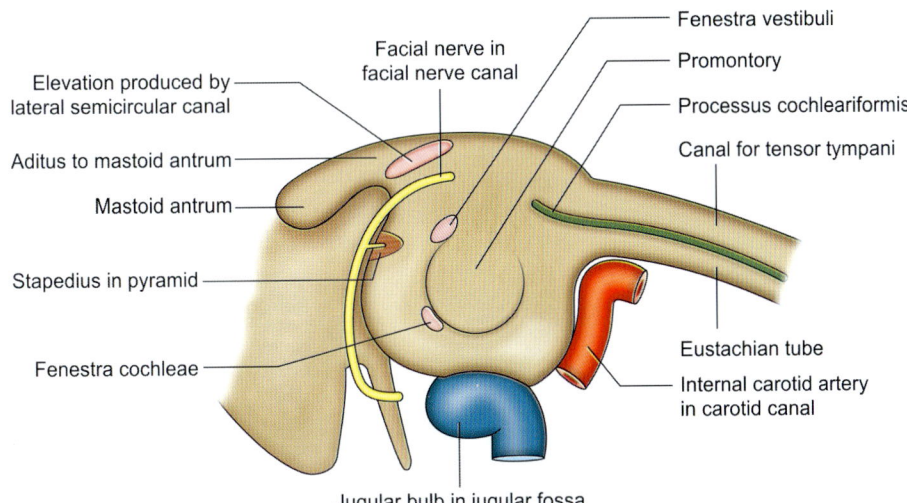

**Fig. 13.9:** Medial wall of middle ear of the right side

6. *Fenestra cochleae* is a rounded opening in the posteroinferior part of the promontory. It connects the tympanic cavity with the scala tympani of the cochlea.

7. Above and posterior to the fenestra vestibuli there is an elevation produced by *facial nerve canal*.

*e. Posterior wall*

1. *Aditus to the mastoid antrum* is an opening in the upper part of posterior wall. It connects epitympanic recess with the mastoid antrum.

2. The medial wall of the aditus to mastoid antrum shows an elevation produced by *lateral semicircular canal*.

3. *Facial nerve canal* lies vertically in the posterior wall anterior to which is a *pyramidal eminence* projecting into the middle ear cavity.

4. Pyramidal eminence is occupied by *stapedius muscle*.

5. *Fossa incudis* is a small depression in the posteroinferior part of the epitympanic recess. It contains short process of incus.

### f. Anterior wall

1. Its lower part is formed by thin plate of bone which separates middle ear from the *carotid canal*.

2. Its upper part is occupied by two openings. Upper opening leads into *canal for tensor tympani*. The lower opening leads into osseous part of *Eustachian tube*. These two canals are visible from the apex side of petrous temporal at petro-squamosal junction.

3. The septum between the aforementioned canals runs on the medial wall and just above the fenestra vestibuli its posterior end curves laterally to form *processus cochleariformis*.

### III. Mastoid antrum

1. It is an air sinus in the petrous part of temporal bone.

2. It is well developed at birth and is almost of adult size.

3. Mastoid antrum is a spherical sinus.

4. In adult the mastoid antrum has a capacity of about 1 ml.

5. *Aditus ad antrum* is an opening in the upper part of anterior wall of mastoid antrum. It connects the antrum with epitympanic recess of middle ear.

6. Roof of antrum is formed by *tegmen tympani*.

7. Posteriorly the antrum is closely related to *sigmoid sinus*.

8. Medial wall is related to posterior *semicircular canal*.

9. Anteroinferiorly the antrum is related to *canal for facial nerve*.

10. Floor has multiple apertures which connect mastoid antrum with *mastoid air cells*.

11. The lateral wall of antrum corresponds to the *suprameatal triangle*. This wall is 1 mm thick at birth and increases at a rate of 1 mm per year until it reaches the adult thickness of about 12.5 mm.

### IV. Mastoid air cells

1. These are very small intercommunicating spaces in the temporal bone continuous with mastoid antrum.

2. At birth neither mastoid air cells nor mastoid process are present. Only after birth mastoid air cells grow out of the mastoid antrum into the mastoid process.

3. The mastoid air cells are mainly seen in the mastoid process, but may extend into the surrounding bones like petrous or squamous parts of temporal bone or even zygomatic bone and jugular process of occipital bone.

4. Some common groups of air cells are as follows (Fig. 13.10):

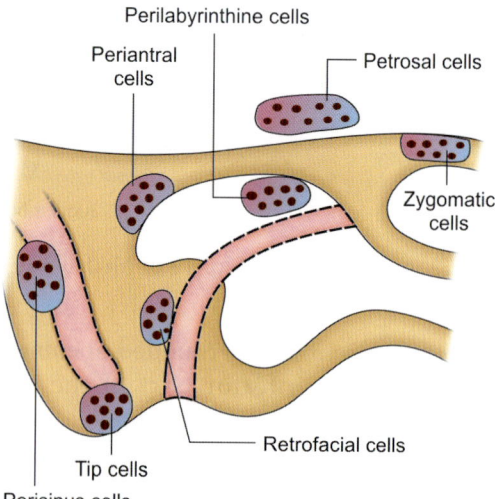

**Fig. 13.10:** Types of air spaces (air cells) in temporal bone

  i. *Tip cells.*

  ii. *Perisinus cells.*

  iii. *Retrofacial cells.*

  iv. *Periantral cells.*

  v. *Perilabyrinthine cells.*

  vi. *Petrous cells.*

  vii. *Zygomatic cells.*

5. Depending upon the pneumatization, the mastoid process may be of three types (Fig. 13.11):

  i. *Pneumatic or cellular.*

  ii. *Sclerotic or acellular.*

  iii. *Diploeic or mixed.*

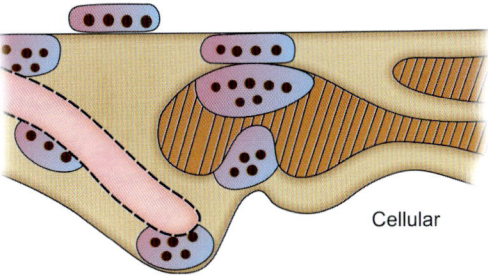

Cellular

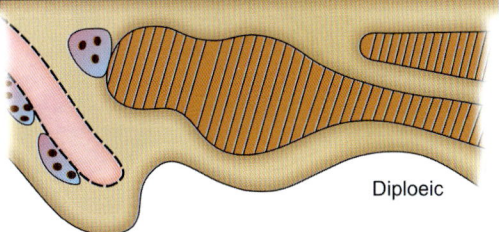

Diploeic

## V. Bony labyrinth (osseous labyrinth) (Figs 13.12 and 13.13)

It consists of three parts, vestibule, semi-circular canals and cochlea.

### A. Vestibule

1. It is the central part of bony labyrinth.

2. In its lateral wall, there is an opening of *fenestra vestibuli* (oval window) occupied by foot plate of stapes in life.

3. Its medial wall corresponds to the fundus of internal acoustic meatus.

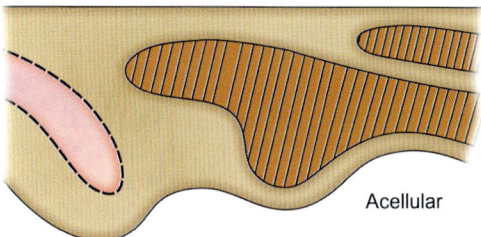

Acellular

**Fig. 13.11:** Types of mastoid

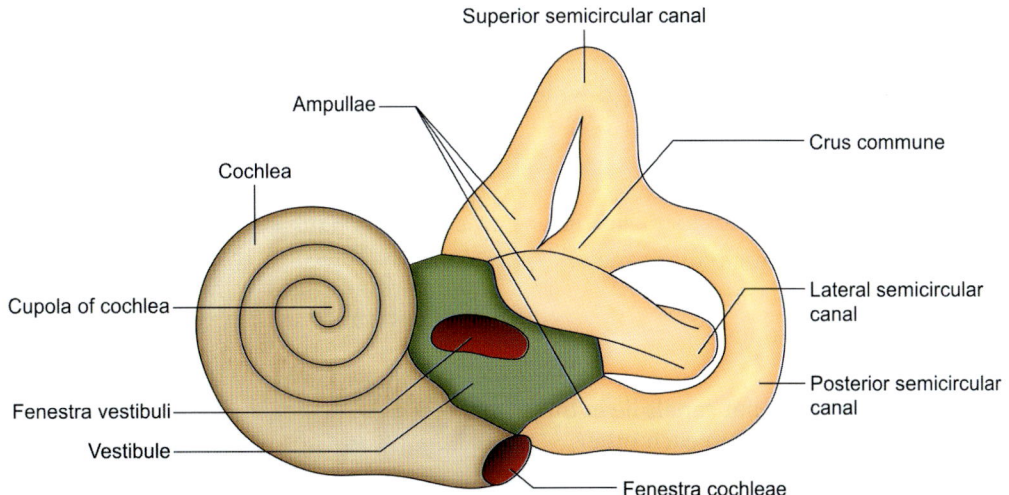

**Fig. 13.12:** Left bony labyrinth: Lateral aspect

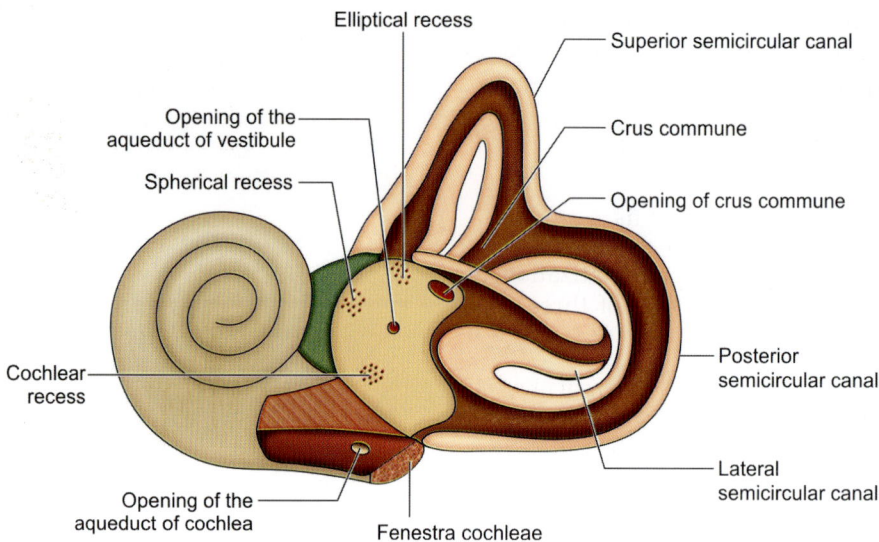

**Fig. 13.13:** The interior of the left osseous labyrinth

4. Anterior part of medial wall has a *spherical recess for saccule*. This recess has multiple perforations which correspond to the openings in inferior vestibular area of fundus of internal acoustic meatus.

5. Posterosuperior to spherical recess is an *elliptical recess* which lodges the *utricle*. This recess also has number of foramina which correspond to openings in the superior vestibular area of fundus.

6. Below the elliptical recess is the opening of aqueduct of vestibule through which passes ductus endolymphaticus.

### B. Semicircular canals

1. They lie posterosuperior to the vestibule.

2. There are three semicircular canals.

   i. Anterior or superior.

   ii. Lateral or horizontal.

   iii. Posterior.

3. Ipsilateral semicircular canals lie in three planes at right angles to each other.

4. Each canal is about two-thirds of a circle.

5. Superior semicircular canal is placed in a vertical plane perpendicular to the long axis of the petrous bone at about 45° with sagittal plane.

6. Posterior semicircular canal is placed in a vertical plane in the long axis of the petrous bone. This also makes an angle of 45° with sagittal plane.

7. Lateral semicircular canal makes an angle of 30° with horizontal plane. This canal lies horizontally if the head is bent forwards for 30°.

8. One end of each canal is dilated called *ampulla*.

9. Both the ends of each canal open into vestibule. Since non-ampullated ends of superior and posterior semicircular canals have common opening in vestibule, thus only five openings connect the three canals with the cavity of the vestibule.

### C. Cochlea

1. It is conical in shape and consists of two and three-quarter spiral turns of a tapering cylindrical canal.

2. The axial bone around which the canal spirals is called *modiolus*.

3. The basal turn of cochlea produces *promontory* on the medial wall of middle ear.

4. From the modiolus a shelf of bone projects into the canal. Since the shelf follows the spiral path of canal, this is called *spiral lamina.*

5. The spiral lamina forms a hook like structure (*called hamulus*) at the apex of modiolus.

6. Basal turn of cochlea shows two holes:

   i. *The fenestra cochleae*

   It is closed in life by *secondary tympanic membrane.*

   ii. *The opening of aqueduct of cochlea*

   It leads downwards to reach the apex of glossopharyngeal notch.

7. Base of modiolus is perforated by spirally arranged foramina. This area corresponds to the cochlear area of the fundus of internal acoustic meatus.

## OSSIFICATION

1. Temporal bone ossifies partly in cartilage and partly in membrane.

2. Squamous and tympanic parts ossify in membrane.

3. Petromastoid part and the styloid process ossify in cartilage.

4. **Appearance of centres**

   i. *Squamous part*

   Single centre appears near the root of zygomatic process during 8th week of intrauterine life.

   ii. *Petromastoid part*

   As many as 14 centres may appear in the cartilaginous mass (otic capsule) around developing internal ear during 5th month of intrauterine life. These centres fuse by 6th month of intrauterine life.

   iii. *Tympanic part*

   Single centre appears during 12th week of intrauterine life. At birth, a tympanic ring represents the tympanic part.

   iv. *Styloid process*

   It develops from cranial end of 2nd arch cartilarge. It ossifies from two centres. Centre for tympanohyal appears before birth and for stylohyal appears after birth.

5. **Fusion**

   i. Squamous part fuses with tympanic part just before birth.

   ii. Petromastoid part fuses with the squamous part and tympanohyal during 1st year.

   iii. Stylohyal fuses with the tympanohyal after puberty.

## APPLIED ANATOMY

1. At birth the tympanic cavity, tympanic membrane, mastoid antrum, ear ossicles and internal ear are all of adult size.

2. At birth the mastoid process is absent and the facial nerve lies on the surface at its exit from stylomastoid foramen. This makes the postauricular incision a risky procedure in newborns.

3. A very long styloid process may lead to multiple complications and in such cases it has to be removed by surgery.

4. In majority of the people the pneumatization of temporal bone is adequate. In 20% cases the pneumatization may be arrested in childhood. This is easily pointed out in X-ray and is called sclerolic or acellular mastoid, a condition which is prone to inflammation.

5. Infections of the middle ear (*otitis media*) invariably leads to the infections of the mastoid antrum and mastoid air cells.

6. Suprameatal triangle is clinically very important as it helps in localizing the mastoid antrum. Mastoid antrum is located 1.25 cm deep to the surface of this triangle.

7. Gross fractures of temporal bones are divided into longitudinal and transverse

in relation to the long axis of petrous temporal bone. Longitudinal fractures are common and are due to blows to the temporal or parietal areas. The transverse fractures are less common and are due to blows in occipital region (Fig. 13.14).

8. Zygomatic arches form the prominences of the face and, therefore, prone to facial injuries.

9. Fracture of zygomatic process of temporal bone may involve the lateral wall of orbit and injure the eye.

10. Squamous part of temporal bone contributes to vault and, therefore, prone to both fissured and depressed fractures. Petrous part contributes to base of skull and thus invariably shows a linear fracture.

11. Fracture of tegmen tympani might connect the subarachnoid space with middle ear leading to CSF leakage into the middle ear. If the tympanic membrane is also damaged then the CSF will appear as discharge through external acoustic meatus. This condition is called *CSF otorrhoea*. The passage may also act as portal for sepsis of meninges and brain.

12. Since the petrous part of temporal bone is very strong, most fracture lines end here without making a tear in it.

13. The indications of the fracture of petrous part of temporal bone are as follows:

    i. CSF otorrhoea.

    ii. Tear of tympanic membrane.

    iii. Collection of blood in the middle ear.

14. Discolouration and edema of the tissue over mastoid process (*Battle's sign*) is indication of sigmoid sinus damage.

15. Fracture of petrous temporal may damage the facial nerve and result into *facial paralysis*.

16. Involvement of vestibulocochlear nerve in petrous fracture will lead to hearing loss, vertigo and nystagmus.

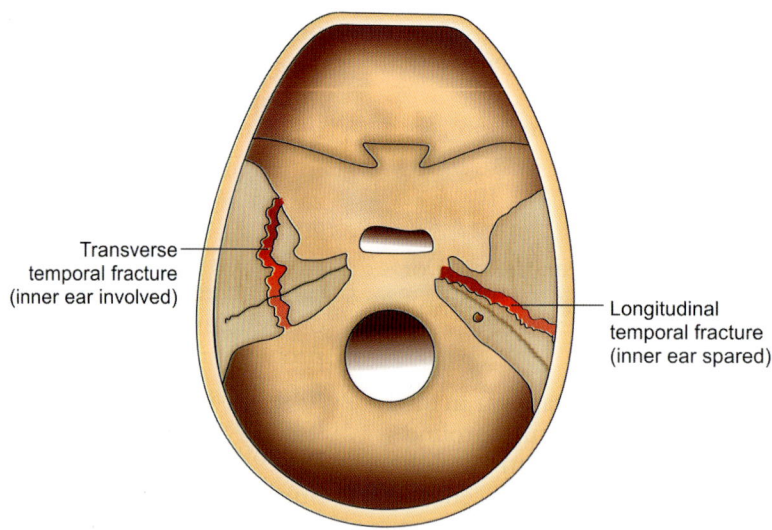

Transverse temporal fracture (inner ear involved)

Longitudinal temporal fracture (inner ear spared)

**Fig. 13.14:** Fractures of temporal bone

# Auditory Ossicles

## TERMINOLOGY

There are three ossicles named malleus, incus and stapes.

These names are Latin in origin, the meanings of which are as follows:

Malleus: Hammer

Incus: An anvil

Stapes: A stirrup

**Note:** *Remember that MIS is situated between tympanic membrane and the oval window where M—Malleus, I—Incus and S—Stapes.*

## FEATURES AND ATTACHMENTS (Fig. 14.1)

### I. Malleus

It consists of head, neck and handle.

#### A. Head

1. It is large upper end of the bone.
2. It is located within the epitympanic recess.
3. Its posterior surface articulates with the body of incus.

#### B. Neck

1. It is the constricted part below the head.
2. Its medial surface is crossed by *chorda tympani nerve*.

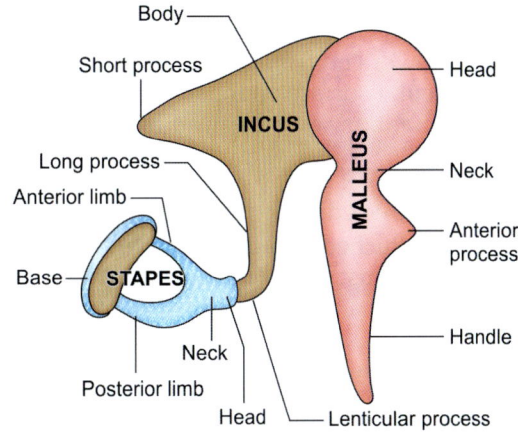

**Fig. 14.1:** Ossicles of the right ear: Lateral aspect

#### C. Handle

1. It is lower elongated part of malleus.
2. It is embedded in the tympanic membrane and moves with it.
3. Its upper end (root) shows following features:
   i. A slight projection on the medial aspect provides attachment to *tendon of tensor tympani*.
   ii. *Anterior process* projects forwards. *Anterior ligament of malleus* is attached to it. This ligament extends into the petrotympanic fissure.

iii. *Lateral process* projects laterally from where extend anterior and posterior malleolar folds to the ends of tympanic sulcus.

## II. Incus

It has a large body and two processes (long and short).

### A. Body

1. It is cubical in shape.
2. Its anterior surface is cancave and articulates with head of malleus.

### B. Processes

#### a. Long process

1. It projects downwards parallel to handle of malleus.
2. Its lower end (*lenticular process*) bears an articular surface on the medial aspect for articulation with the head of stapes.

#### b. Short process

1. It is directed backwards.
2. It is attached by a ligament to the fossa incudis just below the aditus.

## III. Stapes

It has a head, a neck, two limbs (anterior and posterior) and a foot plate (base).

### A. Head

1. It is rounded
2. It articulates with the long process of incus.

### B. Neck

1. It is constricted part adjacent to head.
2. *Tendon of stapedius* is attached to its posterior surface.

### C. Limbs (crura)

1. Anterior and posterior limbs diverges from the neck.
2. These two limbs are attached to the foot plate.

### D. Foot plate (base)

1. It is oval in shape.
2. It fits into the fenestra vestibuli.

## OSSIFICATION

1. Malleus and incus develop from the dorsal end of Meckel's cartilage.
2. Stapes develops from the dorsal end of hyoid arch cartilage.
3. Malleus ossifies by two centres:
   i. One endochondral centre near the neck.
   ii. One centre for anterior process appears in dense connective tissue.
   *Appearance*
   • 4th month of intrauterine life.
   *Fusion*
   • 6th month of intrauterine life.
4. Incus ossifies by single endochondral centre in the upper part of long process. This centre appears at 4th month of intrauterine life.
5. Stapes ossifies by single endochordral centre which appears in the base at 4th month of intrauterine life.
6. At birth the auditory ossicles are of almost adult size.

## FUNCTIONS

1. Malleus functions as a lever as it is attached to the tympanic membrane.
2. The base of stapes is considerably smaller than the tympanic membrane. Due to this fact, the vibratory force of the stapes is about 10 times that of tympanic membrane. Thus the auditory ossicles increase the force but decrease the amplitude of vibrations transmitted from tympanic membrane.

## APPLIED ANATOMY

1. *Treacher Collins syndrome* is a condition in which there are abnormalities of ossicles and

cranio-facial skeleton. This may be one of the causes of congenital conductive deafness.

2. Damage to ossicles in cases of head injury with fracture of temporal bone leads to very severe and permanent *conductive deafness*.

3. Late conductive deafness due to aseptic necrosis of the long process of incus can occur some years after head injury.

4. *Ankylosis of stapes* is a common occurrence in cases of *otosclerosis*.

# 15

# Occipital Bone

## TERMINOLOGY

Word 'occipital' is derived from Greek words 'ob' (meaning back) and 'cipit' (meaning head). Hence referred to the back of head.

## LOCATION

Occipital bone occupies the posterior part of skull and plays major role in the formation of posterior cranial fossa.

## FEATURES AND ATTACHMENTS

The largest foramen of the skull called *foramen magnum*, is located in the occipital bone. The components of occipital bone are better described in relation to this foramen. It consists of 1 *basilar part* (above and in front of foramen magnum), 2 *lateral parts* (lateral to foramen magnum) and 1 *squamous part* (above and behind the foramen magnum).

### I. Foramen magnum

1. It is located in the floor of posterior cranial fossa.
2. It provides a communication between posterior cranial fossa and vertebral canal.
3. Its margins provide attachments to following structures:

   i. Anterior margin: *Anterior atlanto-occipital membrane.*
  ii. Posterior margin: *Posterior atlanto-occipital membrane.*
 iii. Lateral margins: *Alar ligament.*

4. Structures passing through the foramen magnum are as follows:

### A. Anterior part

   i. *Apical ligament of dens.*
  ii. *Superior longitudinal band of cruciform ligament.*
 iii. *Membrana tectoria.*

### B. Posterior part

    i. *Medulla oblongata.*
   ii. *Meninges.*
  iii. *Spinal roots of accessory nerves.*
  iv. *Meningeal branches of upper cervical nerves ($C_{1-3}$)*
   v. *Vertebral arteries.*
  vi. *Sympathetic plexuses around vertebral arteries.*
 vii. *Anterior and posterior spinal arteries.*

### II. Basilar part

It extends upwards and forwards to meet the body of sphenoid. Before 25 years of age a growth cartilage intervenes between sphenoid and basilar part of occipital bone but after this period the two bones fuse. Basilar part has got two surfaces (superior and inferior) and two lateral margins.

### a. Superior surface

1. It is smooth.
2. It forms *clivus* with the body of sphenoid.
3. It is related to *medulla oblongata*.
4. Its lower part receives attachments of following structures from above downwards:
    i. Membrana tectoria.
    ii. Superior longitudinal band of cruciform ligament.
    iii. Apical ligament of dens.
5. Its lateral margins are grooved by *inferior petrosal sinuses*.

### b. Inferior surface

1. Its middle is marked by a tubercle called *pharyngeal tubercle*. This tubercle is approximately 1 cm anterior to foramen magnum. Attached to this tubercle is the upper part of pharyngeal raphe (*pharyngeal ligament*).
2. Anterolateral to pharyngeal tubercle is the area for *longus capitis*.
3. Posterolateral to pharyngeal tubercle (just in front of condyle) is the attachment of *rectus capitis anterior*.

### c. Lateral margins

These are rough and articulate with petrous parts of the temporal bones.

## III. Lateral parts (right and left)

Each can be divided into broader medial portion (adjacent to foramen magnum) and narrower lateral portion (jugular process).

### A. Medial portion

#### a. Inferior surface

1. It is marked by an articular *occipital condyle*.
2. The articular surface of occipital condyle is oval and convex to articulate with concave superior articular process of atlas.
3. Occipital condyle is located lateral to anterior half of foramen magnum.
4. Behind the condyle is *condylar fossa* which may have *condylar canal* for emissary vein from sigmoid sinus.
5. Lateral to anterior part of condyle is the outer opening of *hypoglossal canal*.

#### b. Medial aspect

1. It has got a *tubercle* and a *foramen*.
2. The *tubercle* is situated on the medial aspect of condyle and provides attachment to *alar ligament*.
3. The foramen located just above the tubercle forms the inner opening of *hypoglossal canal*.
4. Following structures pass through hypoglossal canal:
    i. *Hypoglossal nerve.*
    ii. Meningeal branch of ascending pharyngeal artery.

#### c. Superior surface

1. It is marked by an oval eminence called *jugular tubercle.*
2. Jugular tubercle overlies the hypoglossal canal.
3. The posterior part of jugular tubercle often presents a shallow groove for IX, X and XI cranial nerves.

### B. Jugular process

1. Its lateral end presents a rough area which joins the jugular surface of temporal bone by a growth cartilage. The cartilage ossifies at the age of 25 years.
2. Its anterior margin is notched and completes the *jugular foramen* with similar notch on the posterior border of petrous part of temporal bone.
3. Its superior surface is marked by a deep groove which lodges terminal part of *sigmoid sinus*.

4. Its inferior surface provides attachment to *rectus capitis lateralis.*

### IV. Squamous part

It has two surfaces (external and internal), three angles (one superior and two lateral) and four borders (two lambdoid and two mastoid).

### A. Surfaces

#### a. External surface (Figs 15.1 and 15.2)

1. The middle of the external surface is marked by a projection called *external occipital protuberance.*

2. Two lines extend laterally on each side from external occipital protuberance.

   i. A superior faint line is called *highest nuchal line.* This provides attachment to *occipital belly of occipitofrontalis.*

   ii. An inferior well defined line is called *superior nuchal line.* This receives attachments of *trapezius* and *sterno-mastoid* in its medial and lateral parts respectively.

3. A midline ridge extends from the external occipital protuberance to foramen magnum. This is called *external occipital crest.* It gives attachment to *ligamentum nuchae.*

4. Running laterally on each side from the middle of external occipital crest is another ridge called *inferior nuchal line.*

5. There are two muscles attached between superior and inferior nuchal lines on both the sides, i.e. *semispinalis capitis* (medially) and *obliquus capitis superior* (laterally).

6. Similarly, there are two muscles attached to each side of midline below the inferior nuchal line, i.e. *rectus capitis posterior major* (laterally) and *rectus capitis posterior minor* (medially).

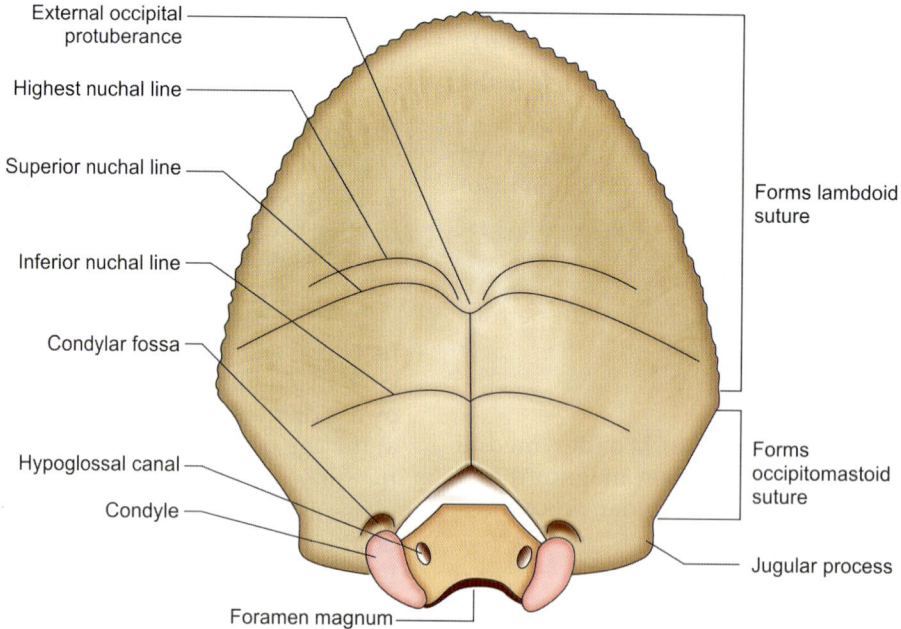

**Fig. 15.1:** Occipital bone: Posterior aspect

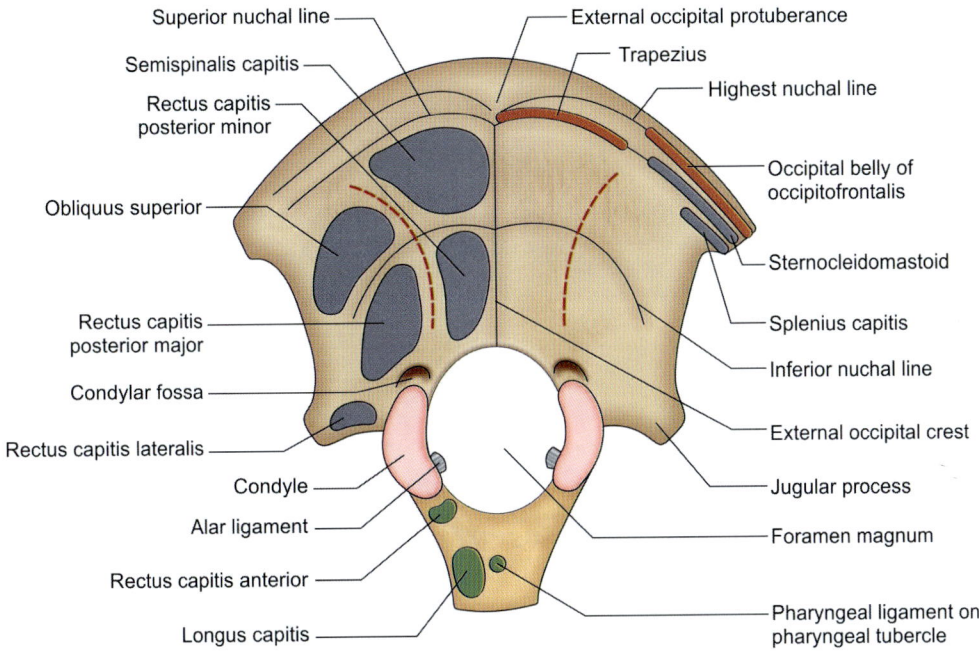

**Fig. 15.2:** Occipital bone: Inferior aspect

**Note:** *Remember that the rectus capitis muscles are named after their relations with occipital condyle. The one lying anterior to condyle is rectus capitis anterior. The muscle lying lateral to condyle is called rectus capitis lateralis. Rectus capitis posterior will naturally be located behind the condyle. Since the latter muscle is two in number, these are further qualified by adding 'major' and 'minor' to their names.*

*It is interesting to note that rectus capitis anterior, lateralis and posterior are attached to three components of occipital bone, i.e. basilar part, lateral part and squamous part respectively.*

### b. Internal surface (Fig. 15.3)

1. Its middle is marked by an elevation called *internal occipital protuberance* which corresponds with the external occipital protuberance on the external surface.
2. Four grooves diverge from the internal occipital protuberance, one upwards, one downwards and two laterally whose margins provide attachments to *falx cerebri, falx cerebelli* and *tentorium cerebelli* respectively.

3. The groove running upwards is produced by *superior sagittal sinus.*

4. The groove running downwards is occupied by *occipital sinus.*

5. The groove extending laterally is produced by corresponding *transverse sinus.*

6. The internal surface is marked by a depression in the midline near the posterior margin of foramen magnum. This is *vermian fossa* related to inferior vermis of cerebellum.

7. Midline elevation extending from internal occipital protuberance to posterior margin of foramen magnum is called *internal occipital crest. Falx cerebelli* is attached to it.

8. On each side of internal occipital crest a hallow is related to *cerebellar hemisphere.*

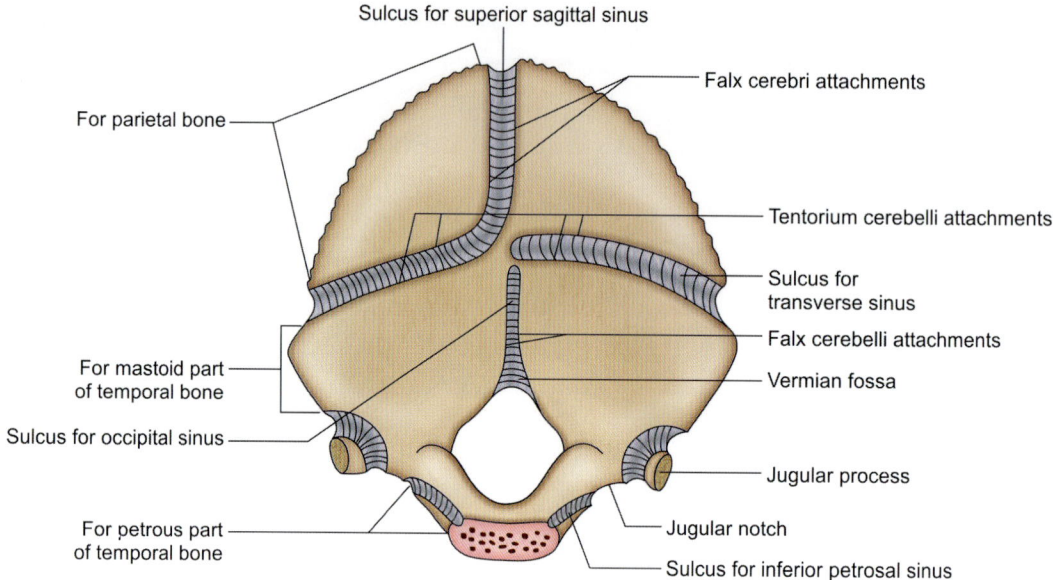

Sulcus for superior sagittal sinus

Falx cerebri attachments

For parietal bone

Tentorium cerebelli attachments

Sulcus for
transverse sinus

Falx cerebelli attachments

For mastoid part
of temporal bone

Vermian fossa

Sulcus for occipital sinus

Jugular process

For petrous part
of temporal bone

Jugular notch

Sulcus for inferior petrosal sinus

**Fig. 15.3:** Occipital bone: Internal aspect

9. Internal surface above the grooves for transverse sinuses is related to *occipital lobes of cerebrum.*

### B. Angles

a. *Superior angle* reaches lambda which during intrauterine life is membranous (*posterior fontanelle*).

b. *Lateral angle* on each side meets with mastoid part of corresponding temporal bone to form *asterion.*

### C. Borders

#### a. Lambdoid border

It extends on each side from superior angle to lateral angle and articulates with posterior margin of corresponding parietal bone to form *lambdoid suture.*

#### b. Mastoid border

It extends on each side from lateral angle to jugular process and articulates with mastoid

part of corresponding temporal bone to form occipitomastoid suture.

### OSSIFICATION

#### I. Origin

1. Part of the occipital bone above the highest nuchal line develops in membrane.
2. Rest of the occipital bone ossifies in cartilage.

#### II. Appearance of centres

Usually seven centres appear at 8th week of intrauterine life as follows:
Four for squamous part (one for each half of the membranous and cartilaginous parts).
Two for lateral parts.
One for basilar part.

#### III. Fusion

1. Membranous and cartilaginous portions fuse with each other when the baby starts holding neck, i.e. 3rd month.

2. Squamous part fuses with lateral parts when primary dentition completes, i.e. at 2 years.

3. Lateral parts fuse with basilar part when the permanent dentition begins, i.e. at 6 years.

4. Basilar part fuses with sphenoid and lateral part fuses with temporal bone at the age of 25 years.

**Note:** *Remember, the occipital condyle is contributed partly from lateral part and partly from basilar part of occipital bone.*

## APPLIED ANATOMY

1. The squamous part of the occipital bone contributing to vault is prone to both fissured and depressed fractures but the portions lying in the base of skull always show linear fracture.

2. Margins of foramen magnum form a natural thick bony buttresses at the base of skull, therefore, the fracture lines often converge towards the foramen magnum.

3. A crack in the inner table of the squamous part of occipital bone may damage the large diploeic vein and produce small *epidural haematoma*.

4. Almost invariably fractures of squamous part of occipital bone in children are associated with rupture of dura mater.

5. Basal fracture of skull involving hypoglossal canal will damage the hypoglossal nerve.

6. A gap in the squamous part of occipital bone forming cranial vault is usually filled with tantalum or titanium due to lack of regeneration in this part whose periosteum is devoid of cambium layer.

# 16

# Zygomatic Bones

## TERMINOLOGY

Term zygomatic is derived from Greek word 'zyg' which means 'yoke'. Hence the zygomatic refers to a bone which is shaped like a yoke uniting the frontal, maxilla and temporal bones.

Zygomatic bone is also called *'malar bone'* because it forms prominence of the cheek which is called 'mala' in Latin.

Term *'zygoma'* is used by clinitians which includes both 'zygomatic bone' and 'zygomatic arch'. Anatomists use the term 'zygoma' for 'zygomatic arch'.

The term *'zygomatic complex'* implies to zygomatic bone and other bones adjacent to it, i.e. maxilla and zygomatic process of frontal bone.

## LOCATION

Zygomatic bones are present in the upper and lateral parts of face.

## FEATURES AND ATTACHMENTS

Each zygomatic bone has three surfaces (lateral, temporal and orbital), five borders (anterosuperior, anteroinferior, posterosuperior, posteroinferior and posteromedial) and two processes (frontal and temporal).

### I. Surfaces

#### A. Lateral surface (Fig. 16.1)

1. It is convex.

2. *Zygomaticofacial foramen* is present near the orbital (anterosuperior) border. It transmits *zygomaticofacial nerve and vessels.*

3. Area below the zygomaticofacial foramen gives origin to two muscles:
   i. *Zygomaticus major* (posteriorly)
   ii. *Zygomaticus minor* (anteriorly).

#### B. Temporal surface (Fig. 16.2)

1. Its anterior part is rough for articulation with maxilla.

2. Its posterior larger part is smooth and forms anterior boundary of temporal fossa.

3. Close to posteroinferior border this surface provides attachment to *masseter muscle.*

4. *Zygomaticotemporal foramen* present on this surface transmits *zygomaticotemporal nerve and vessels.*

#### C. Orbital surface

1. It partly contributes to the lateral wall and floor of the orbit.

2. It possesses *zygomatico-orbital foramina* which transmit:
   i. *Zygomaticotemporal and zygomaticofacial nerves.*
   ii. *Zygomatic branches of lacrimal artery.*

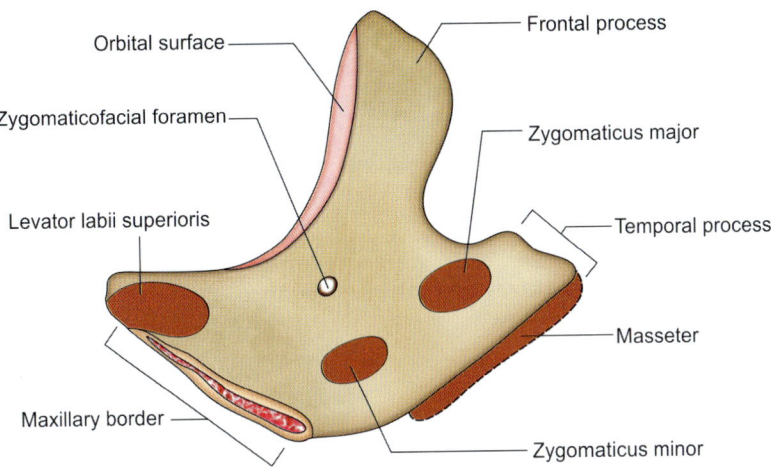

**Fig. 16.1:** Left zygomatic bone: Lateral aspect

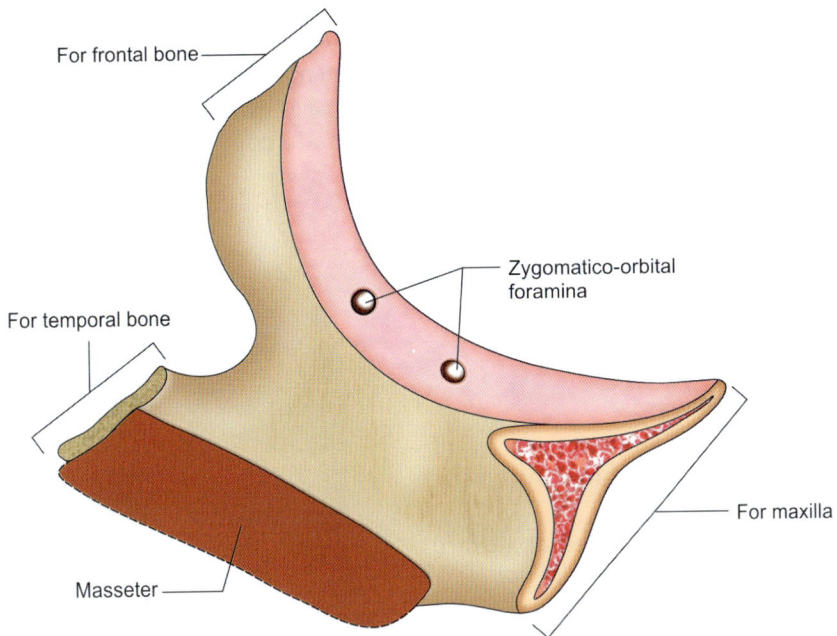

**Fig. 16.2:** Left zygomatic bone: Medial aspect

## II. Borders

### A. Anterosuperior border

1. This is also called *orbital border*.
2. It provides attachement to *orbital septum*.

### B. Anteroinferior border

1. This is also called *maxillary border*.
2. *Levator labii superioris* arises partly from this border near the orbital border.

### C. Posterosuperior border

1. It is also called *temporal border*.
2. *Temporal fascia* is attached to this border.

### D. Posteroinferior border

*Masseter muscle* originates from this border.

### E. Posteromedial border

It articulates with the greater wing of sphenoid above and maxilla below.

### III. Processes

### A. Frontal process

1. It articulates with the zygomatic process of frontal bone (to form *fronto-zygomatic suture*) superiorly and greater wing of sphenoid bone posteriorly.
2. *Whitnall's tubercle* is present on its orbital aspect about 1 cm below the fronto-zygomatic suture. Following structures are attached to this tubercle:
   i. *Lateral check ligament.*
   ii. *Lateral palpebral ligament.*
   iii. *Suspensory ligament of eyeball.*
   iv. *Aponeurosis of levator palpebrae superioris.*

### B. Temporal process

1. It is directed backwards.
2. It articulates with zygomatic process of temporal bone to complete *zygomatic arch*.
3. Its inferior margin and medial surface provide attachment to *masseter muscle*.

### OSSIFICATION

1. Zygomatic bone ossifies in membrane.
2. Usually single centre appears at the age of 8th week of intrauterine life.
3. Sometimes a horizonatal suture divides the bone into an upper larger and a lower smaller segments.

### APPLIED ANATOMY

1. *Malar flush* is the redness of skin over zygomatic prominence. This is observed in tuberculosis, mitral stenosis (narrowing of left atrio-ventricular orifice) and rheumatic fever.
2. Zygomatic bone is of great clinical importance due to its functional significance
   i. It protects the globe of eye.
   ii. It gives origin to masseter muscle.
   iii. It transmits part of the masticatory forces to cranium
   iv. It absorbs the force of an impact before it reaches the brain.
3. When a rapidly moving object hits the zygomatic bone, a comminuted fracture results with displacement of bone fragments (Fig. 16.3).
4. *Tripod* fracture means fracture of zygomatic complex. Zygomatic bone is like

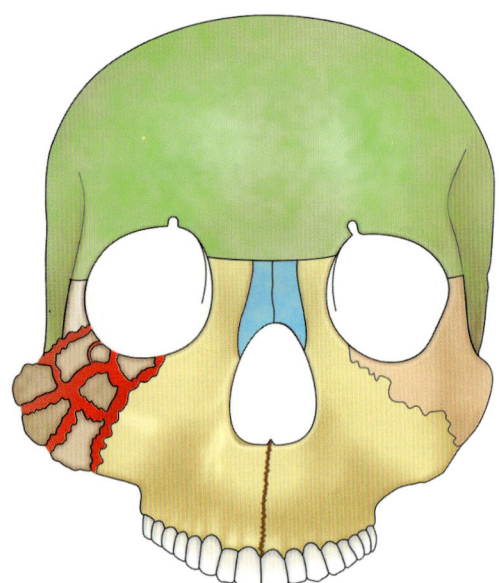

**Fig. 16.3:** Comminuted fracture of body of zygomatic bone and orbital floor

three legged stool, the seat of stool is main portion of zygomatic bone while legs are frontal process, inferior orbital margin and zygomatic buttress.

5. Frontozygomatic suture, zygomatic prominence, the zygomatic buttress and 1st molar tooth, all lie in same vertical line. In majority of the cases, zygomatic complex fracture is associated with rotation along this axis (Fig. 16.4).

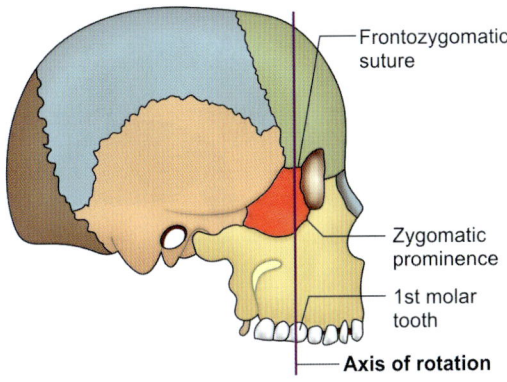

**Fig. 16.4:** Vertical axis of rotation during zygomatic complex fracture

6. Zygomatic bone forms one of the principal means by which occlusal stress is transmitted from the maxilla and spreads over the base of skull.

7. *Fracture of zygoma* (zygomatic arch and zygomatic bone) is second among the common fractures of the middle 3rd of the face.

8. The junctions of frontal and temporal processes of zygomatic bone form important landmarks in the treatment of maxillo-facial injuries.

9. The periosteum and attachment of strong temporal fascia limit the displacement of zygomatic bone following injury.

10. In *depressed fracture of zygomaticomaxillary complex*, there is displacement of zygomatic bone without its fracture (Fig. 16.5).

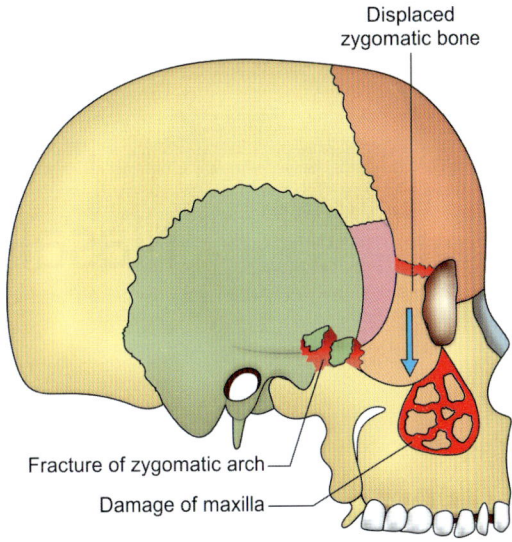

**Fig. 16.5:** Depressed fracture of zygomatico-maxillary complex

11. *Le Fort III fracture* of face is a horizontal fracture just below the base of skull. The fracture line passes laterally through frontozygomatic sutures. As there is a concurrent fracture of zygomatic arches, the maxillae and zygomatic bones are separated from rest of the skull (Fig. 16.6).

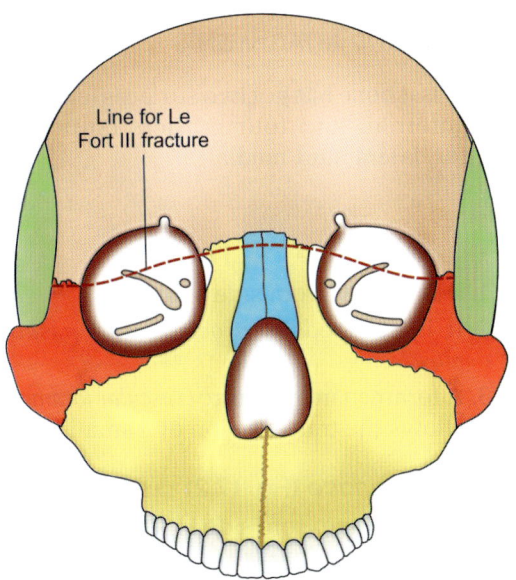

**Fig. 16.6:** Le Fort III fracture

# Nasal Bones

## TERMINOLOGY

Nasal bone is so named because of its location. It forms the bridge of the nose.

## LOCATION

Two nasal bones meet with each other in midline in the upper part of external nose. They are located below the nasal part of frontal bone and between the frontal processes of maxillae.

## FEATURES AND ATTACHMENTS

Each nasal bone has got two surfaces (external and internal) and four borders (superior, inferior, lateral and medial).

### I. Surfaces

#### A. External surface (Fig. 17.1)

1. It is convex from side to side.
2. It is covered by *procerus* and *nasalis muscles*.
3. A foramen in the centre (*vascular foramen*) allows the transmission of a small vein.

#### B. Internal surface (Fig. 17.2)

1. It is concave from side to side
2. It presents a *vertical groove* for the *anterior ethmoidal nerve*.

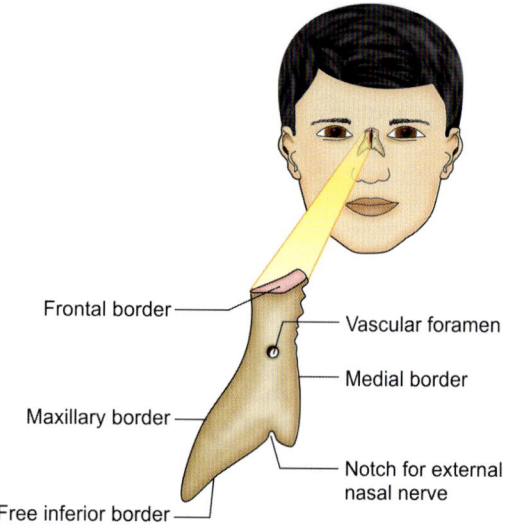

Fig. 17.1: Right nasal bone: External surface

### II. Borders

#### A. Superior border

1. It is serrated.
2. It articulates with nasal part of frontal bone.

#### B. Inferior border

1. It is notched for the passage of *external nasal nerve*.
2. It is continuous with the lateral nasal cartilage.

120

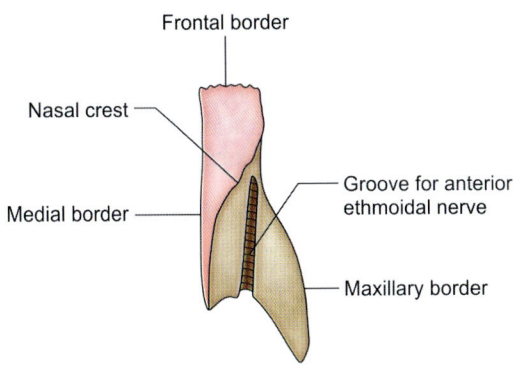

**Fig. 17.2:** Right nasal bone: Internal surface

### C. Lateral border

It articulates with frontal process of maxilla.

### D. Medial border

1. It is thick above than below.
2. It articulates with opposite nasal bone (*to form internasal suture*) and prolonged behind as *nasal crest*.
3. Nasal crest articulates with following structures from above downwards:

   i. *Nasal spine of frontal bone.*

   ii. *Perpendicular plate of ethmoid.*

   iii. *Septal cartilage.*

### OSSIFICATION

1. Nasal bone ossifies in membrane overlying the anterior part of cartilaginous nasal capsule
2. Centre of ossification appears in its middle during 3rd month of intrauterine life.

### APPLIED ANATOMY

1. Nasal bone is usually fractured due to direct hard blow.
2. The *fractures of nasal bone* are transverse in nature.
3. The common site for the fracture of nasal bone is half (½) inch above its inferior border.
4. Slight mobility of anteroinferior part of the nasal bone protects the nose against mild injuries.
5. An impact directed in the anteroposterior plane will cause a depression of the nasal bridge due to fracture of nasal bone, frontal process of maxilla and septal cartilage.

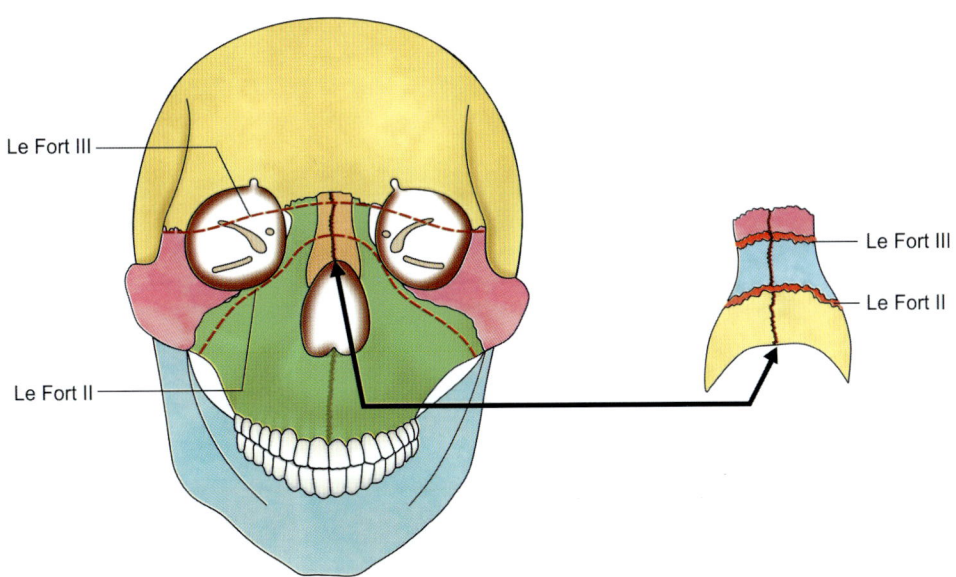

**Fig. 17.3:** Le Fort fractures

6. A force directed from the lateral aspect will result in a deviation of the nasal bridge to opposite side.

7. Traumatic alteration in the shape of nose because of fracture of nasal bones is of great clinical importance due to cosmetic reasons specially in young females.

8. In cases of *Le Fort II and Le Fort III fractures* of maxillae, nasal bones are also involved. Le Fort I fracture of maxillae spares the nasal bone.

# 18

# Lacrimal Bones

## TERMINOLOGY

'Lacrimal' is a Latin word which means 'tear'. The bone is so named because of its relation with the tear sac.

## PECULIARITIES

1. It is most fragile amongst the cranial bones.
2. It is the smallest of the cranial bones.

## LOCATION

1. There are two lacrimal bones.
2. Each lacrimal bone is located in the anterior part of the medial wall of orbit.
3. It also contributes to the middle meatus of nose.

## FEATURES AND ATTACHMENTS

Lacrimal bone is rectangular in shape. It has two *surfaces* (*medial and lateral*) and four *borders* (*anterior, posterior, superior and inferior*).

### I. Surfaces
### A. Medial surface (Fig. 18.1)

1. It is also called nasal surface.
2. Its anteroinferior part contributes partly to the middle meatus of nose.

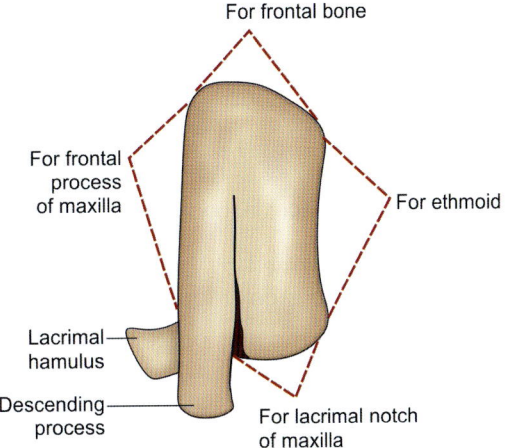

**Fig. 18.1:** Right lacrimal bone: Medial surface

3. Its posterosuperior part articulates with the ethmoid and completes few anterior ethmoidal air cells.

### B. Lateral surface (Fig. 18.2)

1. It is also known as the orbital surface.
2. It is divided into anterior and posterior parts by a vertical crest called *posterior lacrimal crest*.
3. The anterior part is grooved and forms posterior half of the floor of the *lacrimal groove*. Anterior half of the lacrimal

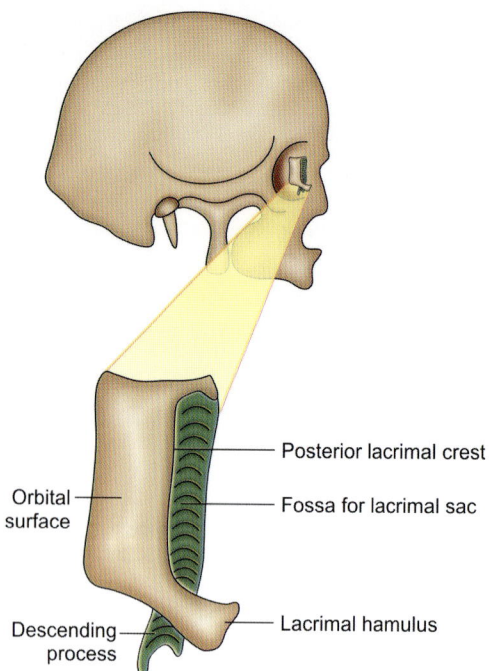

**Fig. 18.2:** Right lacrimal bone: Lateral surface

groove is formed by frontal process of maxilla. The groove lodges *lacrimal sac*.

4. Portion behind the posterior lacrimal crest is smooth and forms part of medial wall of orbit.

5. Lower end of posterior lacrimal crest projects forwards as *lacrimal hamulus*. It articulates with maxilla to complete the *upper end of nasolacrimal canal*.

6. Posterior lacrimal crest provides attachment to *lacrimal fascia*.

7. The crest and small area of lateral surface immediately behind it give origin to *lacrimal part of orbicularis oculi muscle*.

8. The medial wall of groove projects downwards as *descending process*. This process articulates with the lips of nasolacrimal groove of the maxilla and lacrimal process of inferior concha to complete the bony canal for nasolacrimal duct.

## II. Borders

### A. Anterior border

It articulates with the frontal process of maxilla.

### B. Posterior border

It articulates with the orbital plate of ethmoid.

### C. Superior border

It articulates with the nasal notch of frontal bone.

### D. Inferior border

It articulates with the orbital surface of maxilla.

## OSSIFICATION

1. Lacrimal bone ossifies in membrane.
2. Single centre of ossification appears in the mesenchyme around the cartilaginous nasal capsule.
3. The centre appears at about 12th week of intrauterine life.

## APPLIED ANATOMY

1. A severe impact on the nasal bridge may involve the lacrimal bone and damage the lacrimal passage.
2. Lacrimal bone is included by clinicians in the central portion of middle 3rd facial skeleton. All the bones of middle 3rd facial skeleton receive adequate blood supply from periosteal arteries and, therefore, all the fragments of fractured bone retain a periosteal blood supply.
3. Lacrimal bone is involved in *Le Fort III fracture*.
4. Since the anteroinferior part of nasal surface of lacrimal bone is covered with nasal mucosa, the fracture of the bone may open into nasal cavity with potential risk of infection.
5. To reach the medial wall of optic canal during surgical procedure called *optic nerve*

*decompression*, most of the bones of medial wall of orbit (including lacrimal bone) are infractured.

6. Lacrimal bone is very fragile, therefore an extraprecaution should be taken to avoid trauma during surgery of lacrimal system.

7. In some of the cases of obstruction of lacrimal sac or nasolacrimal duct, *dacryocystorhinostomy* is performed. In this operation an artificial passage is made for drainage into nasal cavity, by breaking the lacrimal bone.

# Ethmoid Bone

## TERMINOLOGY

'Ethmoid' is a Greek word which means 'sieve like'. Ethmoid is so named because it possesses a perforated (sieve like) plate called cribriform plate.

## LOCATION

Single ethmoid bone is situated in the anterior part of the base of the cranium between the orbits. It forms part of the medial wall of the orbits and part of the bony septum, roofs and lateral walls of the nasal cavities.

## FEATURES AND ATTACHMENTS

Ethmoid bone consists of a *cribriform plate*, a *perpendicular* plate and two lateral masses called *labyrinths*.

## I. Cribriform plate (Fig. 19.1)

1. It is the median part of the superior surface of ethmoid.
2. It contributes to the median portion of anterior cranial fossa (anterior part of the interior of base of skull).
3. It occupies the ethmoidal notch of the frontal bone.
4. It possesses a median triangular upward projection called *crista galli* (named because

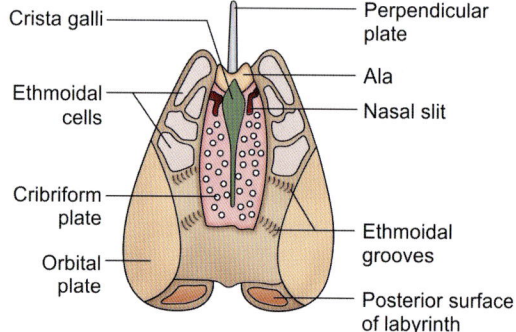

Fig. 19.1: Ethmoid: Superior aspect

of its resemblance to crown of a cock, zoological name of which is *Gallus domesticus*).
5. Posterior sloping border of the crista galli gives attachment to *falx cerebri*.
6. Anterior border of the crista galli has two alae which articulate with frontal bone to complete *foramen caecum. Emissary vein* passes through this foramen.
7. On each side of the crista galli, the cribriform plate shows a number of perforations through which pass about *15–20 filaments of the olfactory nerve*. This part is also related to olfactory bulb superiorly.
8. Just lateral to anterior part of crista galli there is a slit like passage for a *process of dura mater*.

9. Just lateral to the anterior end of slit there is a foramen for the passage of *anterior ethmoidal nerve.*

## II. Perpendicular plate (Fig. 19.2)

1. It is a quadrangular flat plate projecting downwards from the midline of cribriform plate.
2. Its anterior border articulates with the nasal process of frontal bone and the crest of the nasal bones.
3. Its posterior border articulates with sphenoidal crest above and vomer below.
4. Its superior border is attached to the cribriform plate.
5. Its inferior border receives the attachment of septal cartilage.
6. Its surfaces are mainly smooth except in the upper parts where there are grooves for filaments of olfactory nerves.

## III. Labyrinths

Large number of air filled spaces (*ethmoidal air cells*) constitute the labyrinth. These air cells are divisible into anterior, middle and posterior *ethmoidal sinuses* by bony plates. Many of these air cells open on the surface and completed only when articulating with the adjacent bones. Each labyrinth may be considered to have six surfaces.

### A. Upper surface

1. It has several open air cells which are completed only after articulation with edges of ethmoidal notch.
2. It has two grooves which are converted into anterior and posterior ethmoidal canals by articulation with frontal bone.

### B. Lower surface

It articulates with upper part of the nasal surface of maxilla to complete the ethmoidal air cells from below.

### C. Anterior surface

It possesses half cut air sinuses which are completed by the frontal process of maxilla and lacrimal bone.

### D. Posterior surface (Fig. 19.3)

It articulates with sphenoidal concha and orbital process of palatine bone to complete the posterior ethmoidal sinus.

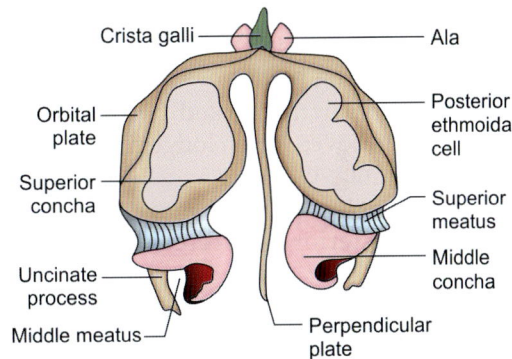

**Fig. 19.3:** Ethmoid: Posterior aspect

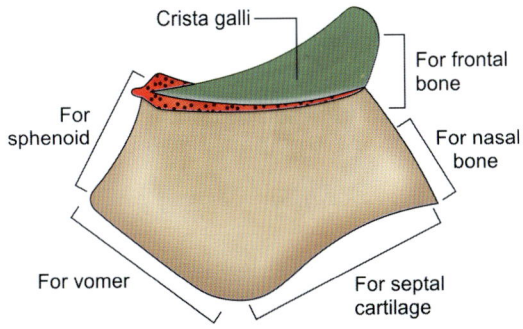

**Fig. 19.2:** Perpendicular plate of ethmoid: Right lateral aspect

### E. Lateral surface (Fig. 19.4)

1. It is thin and smooth plate called *orbital plate.*
2. It covers the middle and posterior ethmoidal sinuses.
3. It forms large part of medial wall of orbit.
4. It is quadrangular in shape and articulates as follows:

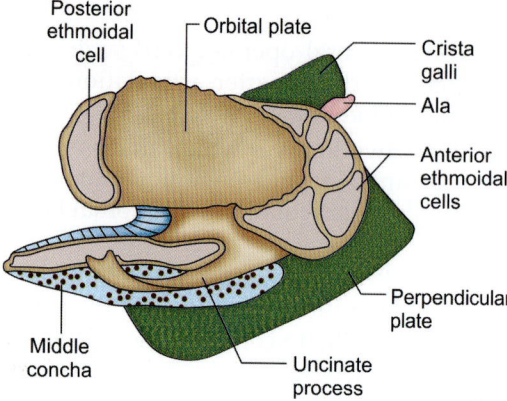

**Fig. 19.4:** Ethmoid: Right lateral aspect

   i. Superiorly with orbital plate of frontal bone.

   ii. Inferiorly with the maxilla and orbital process of palatine bone.

   iii. Anteriorly with lacrimal bone.

   iv. Posteriorly with sphenoid bone.

### F. Medial surface

1. It forms part of the lateral wall of corresponding half of nasal cavity.

2. Its upper part is marked by numerous vertical grooves which lodge filaments of olfactory nerve.

3. Its posterior part is marked by an anteroposterior fissure called *superior meatus*.

4. Posterior ethmoidal sinus opens into superior meatus.

5. Superior meatus is bounded above by a curved plate called *superior nasal concha*.

6. Below and in front of superior meatus is another curved plate of bone called *middle nasal concha*.

7. Lateral surface of middle concha is concave and forms medial wall of *middle meatus*.

8. Lateral wall of middle meatus is marked by a swelling produced by middle ethmoidal air cells. This swelling is called *bulla ethmoidalis*.

9. Middle ethmoidal sinus opens on the surface of bulla or immediately above it.

10. A thin bar of bone called *uncinate process* projects downwards and backwards from the anterior part of the labyrinth.

11. The curved gap between uncinate process and bulla is called *hiatus semilunaris*.

12. The upper end of hiatus semilunaris is continuous with a curved canal called *ethmoidal infundibulum*.

13. Anterior ethmoidal sinus opens into the infundibulum.

14. In 50% cases the infundibulum continues superiorly as *frontonasal duct* to reach the frontal sinus.

### OSSIFICATION

1. At the age of 3rd month of intrauterine life the walls of nasal cavity are marked by a cartilaginous framework called *cartilaginous nasal capsule*.

2. Cartilaginous nasal capsule consists of two lateral regions and a median nasal part.

3. Single centre appears for each labyrinth in the lateral region of nasal capsule at about 5th month of intrauterine life.

4. Perpendicular plate and crista galli ossify from single centre which appears in the median septal part of nasal capsule at the age of 1st year after birth.

5. The labyrinths fuse with perpendicular plate in the region of cribriform plate at about 2 years of age.

6. The ethmoid air cells begin to develop during intrauterine life and are present in the form of narrow pouches at birth.

### APPLIED ANATOMY

1. A severe impact on the nasal bridge may involve frontal processes of maxillae and two orbital plates of ethmoid bones.

2. In case of head injury, a discharge of CSF from nose (*CSF rhinorrhoea*) is indicative of

fracture of cribriform plate of ethmoid in the anterior cranial fossa.

3. If the basilar fracture involves the cribriform plate, it may result into *anosmia* (loss of smell sensation) due to damage of olfactory nerve filaments.

4. *Fracture of cribriform plates* may cause meningitis if it opens into the nasal cavity.

5. Bony septum of nose (perpendicular plate of ethmoid and vomer) is paper thin and does not resist much to forces responsible for fracture.

6. The ethmoid is *spared in Le Fort I fracture* while *involved in Le Fort II and III fractures* (Fig. 19.5).

7. Since the ethmoid bone is clothed in mucosa over large areas of its surfaces, its fractures open into nasal cavity or ethmoid air cells with potential risk of infection.

8. *Nasal ethmoidostomy* is performed in several operations involving the ethmoidal labyrinth. In this an artificial opening is made in the ethmoidal labyrinth to drain the sinuses, e.g. after removal of frontoethmoidal mucoceles or optic nerve decompression in optic canal.

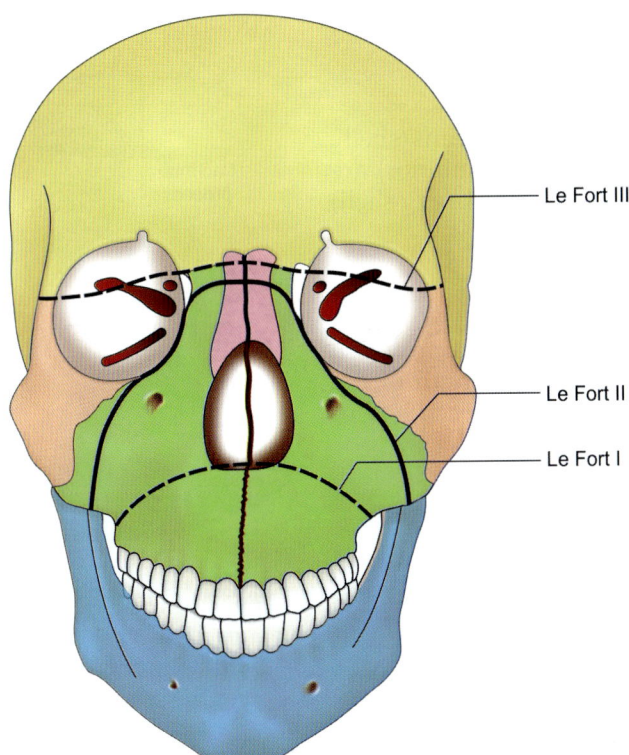

**Fig. 19.5:** Common fractures of maxillae and other bones of skull

# Inferior Nasal Conchae

## TERMINOLOGY

'Concha' is a Latin word which means 'shell'. Conchae (superior, middle and inferior) are bracket like projections of thin (like egg shell) bones from lateral wall of nose.

## LOCATION

Inferior concha is an independent bone whose long axis occupies the whole length of the lower part of the lateral wall of each half of nasal cavity.

## FEATURES AND ATTACHMENTS

Each inferior concha has two *ends* (*anterior and posterior*), two *surfaces* (*medial and lateral*) and two *borders* (*superior and inferior*).

### I. Ends

#### A. Anterior end

It is pointed and directed forwards.

#### B. Posterior end

It directed backwards and is more pointed and tapering.

### II. Surfaces

#### A. Medial surface (Fig. 20.1)

1. It is convex.

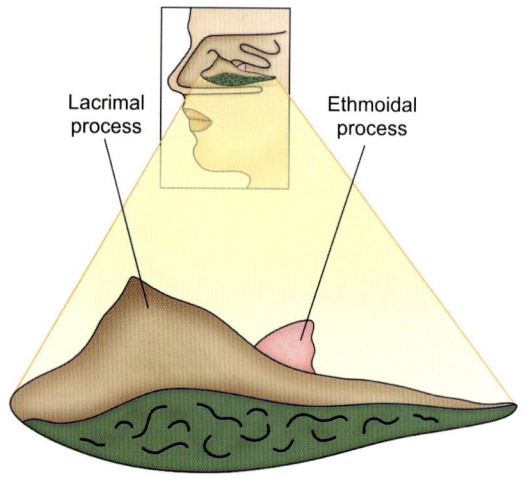

**Fig. 20.1:** Right inferior concha: Medial aspect

Lacrimal process

Ethmoidal process

2. It has numerous apertures and grooves for vessels.

#### B. Lateral surface (Fig. 20.2)

1. It is concave.
2. It forms medial wall of the inferior meatus of nose.

### III. Borders

#### A. Superior border

1. It is thin and irregular.
2. It is divided into three parts:

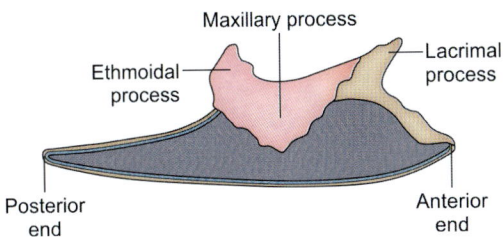

**Fig. 20.2:** Right inferior concha: Lateral aspect

### a. Anterior part

This articulates with conchal crest of maxilla.

### b. Posterior part

This articulates with conchal crest of palatine bone.

### c. Middle region

This part possesses three processes which are as follows from anterior to posterior:

*i. Lacrimal process*

It is an upward projection to articulate with the descending process of lacrimal bone.

*ii. Maxillary process*

It is a curved downward projection which articulates with nasal surface of maxilla and lower part of anterior border of perpendicular plate of palatine bone.

*iii. Ethmoidal process*

It is an upward projection to articulate with uncinate process of ethmoid.

### B. Inferior border

1. It is free.
2. It is thick.

## OSSIFICATION

1. It develops from the lowest part of lateral region of the cartilaginous nasal capsule.
2. The centre of ossification appears during the 5th month of intrauterine life.

## APPLIED ANATOMY

1. Inferior nasal concha is at great risk in cases of *mid-facial injuries*.
2. Inferior concha receives adequate blood supply from periosteal arteries and, therefore, all the fragments of the fractured bone retain a periosteal blood supply.
3. Inferior concha is clothed in nasal mucosa over large areas of its surfaces and, therefore, the fractures usually open to the nasal cavity with potential risk of infection.
4. *Infracture of the inferior concha* is some times needed during management of congenital lacrimal defects (Fig. 20.3).

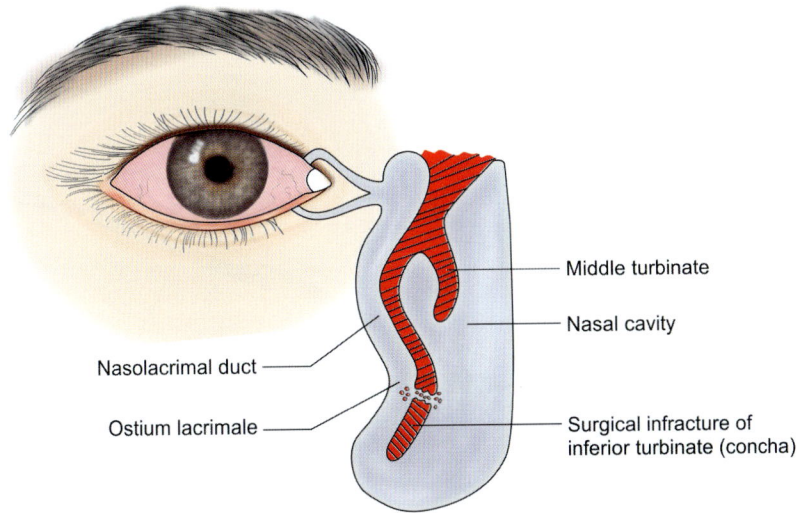

**Fig. 20.3:** Infracture of inferior concha (turbinate)

# 21

# Vomer

## TERMINOLOGY

'Vomer' is a Latin word. The term is used for the thin plate of bone between the nostrils.

## LOCATION

Vomer forms the posteroinferior part of the septum of nose (Fig. 21.1).

## FEATURES AND ATTACHMENTS

Vomer has got two *surfaces* (*right and left*) and four *borders* (*superior, inferior, anterior and posterior*).

## I. Surfaces

1. It has small grooves for vessels.
2. A large groove runs downwards and forwards. This is meant for *nasopalatine nerve and vessels*.

## II. Borders

### A. Superior border

1. It is thick.
2. Two lateral projections (*alae*) enclose a deep furrow which fits over the rostrum of sphenoid.

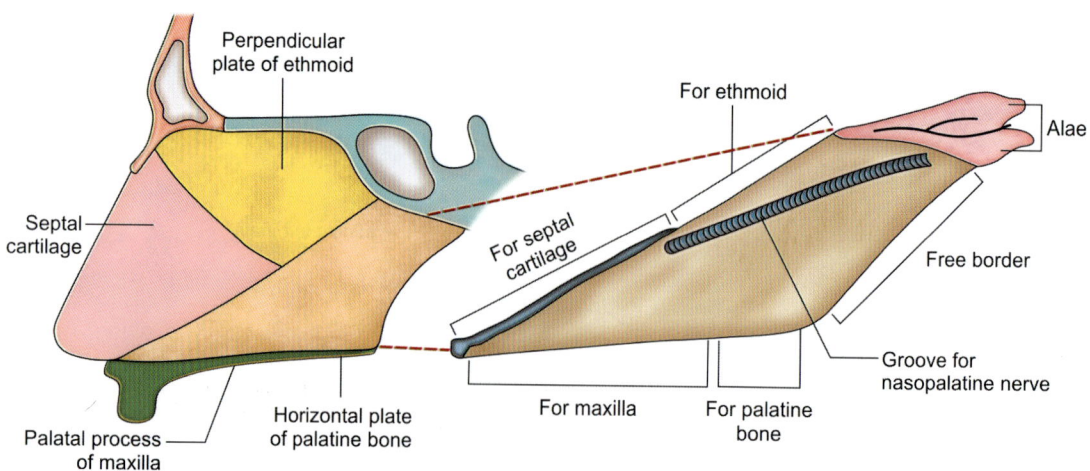

**Fig. 21.1:** Vomer: Left view

3. The margin of ala intervenes between body of sphenoid and vaginal process of medial pterygoid plate. Under surface of the ala forms *vomerovaginal canal* with vaginal process (Fig. 21.2).

### B. Inferior border

It articulates with nasal crest formed by the maxillae and palatine bones.

### C. Anterior border

1. It is the longest border.
2. Its upper half articulates with the posterior border of the perpendicular plate of ethmoid bone.
3. Its lower half is attached to septal cartilage.

### D. Posterior border

1. It is free.
2. It is situated between two posterior nasal apertures (*choanae*).

## OSSIFICATION

1. Vomer develops by ossification of membrane covering the me dian septal part of the cartilaginous nasal capsule.
2. One centre of ossification appears on each side of the cartilage at about 8th week of intrauterine life. giving rise to two bony plates separated by a cartilage.
3. Two bony plates fuse with each other in the lower part at about 12th week of intrauterine life.
4. The cartilaginous plate is gradually absorbed allowing the fusion of two bony plates which proceeds upwards from below. Fusion is completed at puberty.

## APPLIED ANATOMY

1. Vomer is paper thin and does not resist much to forces responsible for fracture.
2. Vomer is involved in all three types of *Le Fort fractures* of mid-facial skeleton (Fig. 21.3).

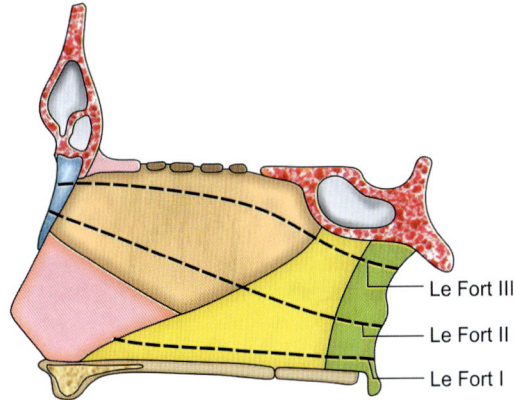

**Fig. 21.3:** Le Fort fractures

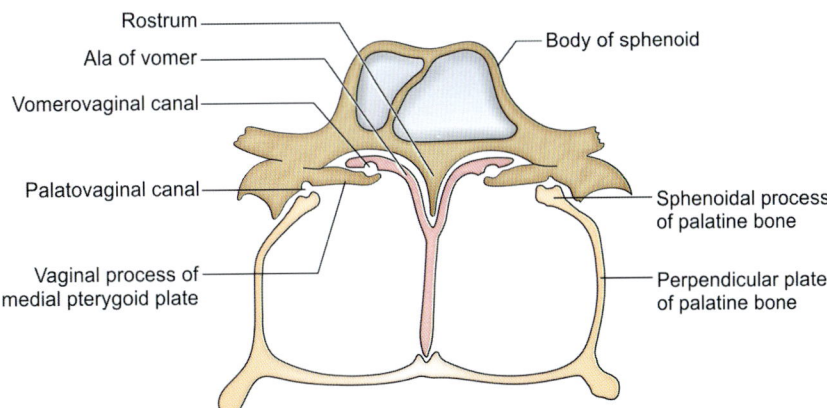

**Fig. 21.2:** Vomerovaginal and palatovaginal canals

3. Vomer receives adequate blood supply from periosteal arteries and therefore all the fragments of fractured bone retain a periosteal blood supply.

4. A transverse fracture of vomer due to direct blow on the nose, can lead to *deviation of nasal septum (DNS)*.

5. Vomer is clothed in mucosa over large areas of its surfaces, and therefore, its fracture opens into nasal cavity with potential risk of infection.

6. Vomer may be deviated from the median plane as a result of birth injury or a congenital malformation.

7. In case of severe deviation, nasal septum comes into contact with the lateral wall of the nasal cavity. Surgical repair *(submucosal resection—SMR)* is usually necessary to correct the deviation.

# 22

# Sphenoid Bone

## TERMINOLOGY

'Sphenoid' is derived from Greek word 'sphen' which means 'a wedge'. The bone is so named because it is wedged between the frontal bone in front and occipital bone behind.

## ANATOMICAL POSITION

1. Hypophyseal fossa faces upwards.
2. Pterygoid processes descend vertically downwards.
3. Openings of sphenoidal sinuses are directed forwards.

## ARTICULATIONS

Sphenoid is a key bone in the cranial skeleton as it articulates with following eight bones:

1. *Frontal*
2. *Parietal*
3. *Temporal*
4. *Occipital*
5. *Vomer*
6. *Zygomatic*
7. *Palatine*
8. *Ethmoid*

## SHAPE

Sphenoid resembles a 'bat' with its wings stretched out.

## FEATURES AND ATTACHMENTS

Sphenoid consists of a central *body*, four *wings* (*two greater and two lesser*) and two *pterygoid processes (right and left)*.

### I. Body

It has six surfaces (superior, inferior, anterior, posterior and two lateral) and a pair of air filled cavities (sphenoidal sinuses).

#### A. Surfaces

##### a. Superior (cerebral) surface (Fig. 22.1)

It shows of following features from anterior to posterior.

  i. *Jugum sphenoidale*
   1. It is smooth.
   2. It articulates with posterior margin of cribriform plate.
   3. It is related on each side to gyrus rectus of cerebral hemisphere and olfactory tract.
  ii. *Sulcus chiasmatis*
   1. It is a transverse groove behind the jugum sphenoidale.

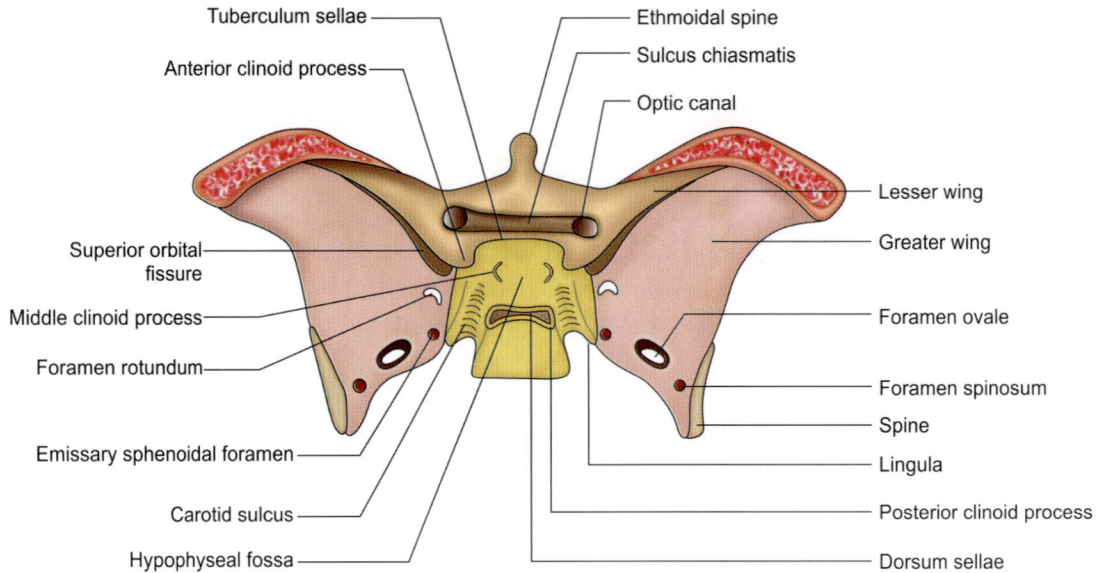

**Fig. 22.1:** Sphenoid bone: Superior aspect

2. *Optic chiasma* lies just above it.

3. It leads laterally into *optic canal*.

iii. *Tuberculum sellae*

It is an elevation just behind the sulcus chiasmatis.

iv. *Sella turcica*

1. It is a depressed area behind the tuberculum sellae.

2. *Hypophyseal fossa* is the deepest part of the sella turcica. It lodges *pituitary gland*.

3. Anterior part of sella turcica is bounded on each side by an elevation called *middle clinoid process*.

v. *Dorsum sellae*

It is a square plate of bone behind the sella turcica.

vi. *Posterior clinoid process*

1. Superior angles of dorsum sellae project laterally into *posterior clinoid processes*.

2. Attached margin of *tentorium cerebelli* is attached to this process on each side.

vii. *Upper part of clivus*

1. It is sloping behind the dorsum sellae.

2. It is formed by the posterior parts of body and dorsum sellae.

3. It supports the pons.

b. *Posterior surface* (Fig. 22.2)

1. It is rough.

2. It articulates with the basilar part of occipital bone.

c. *Anterior and inferior surfaces* (Fig. 22.3)

1. Midline of the anterior surface is marked by a triangular crest called *sphenoidal crest*.

2. Sphenoidal crest articulates with the upper part of the posterior border of perpendicular plate of ethmoid.

3. The midline of the inferior surface is marked by a triangular spine called *sphenoidal rostrum*. It fits into the groove between the alae of vomer.

4. Both anterior and inferior surfaces of the body on either side of midline, are

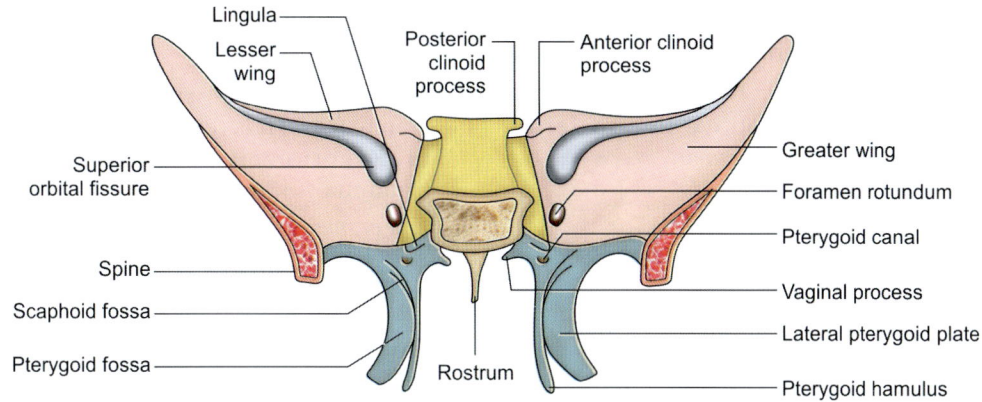

**Fig. 22.2:** Sphenoid bone: Posterior aspect

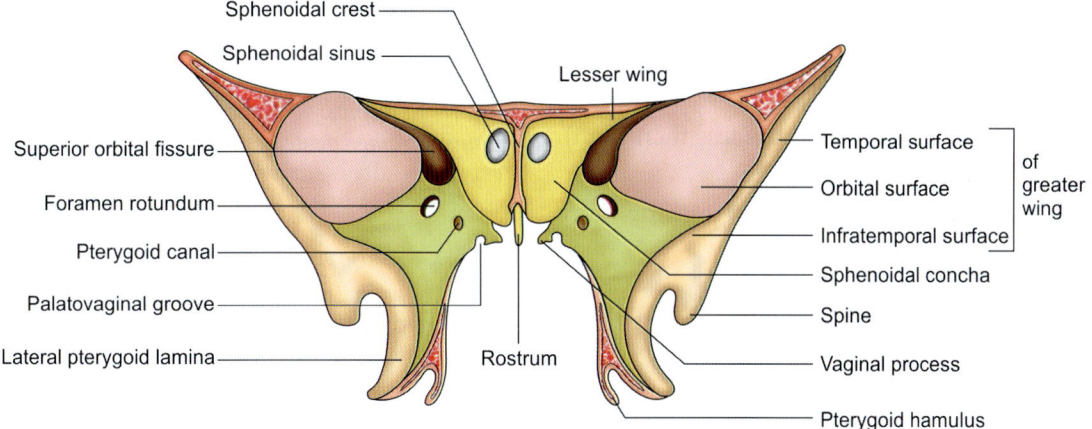

**Fig. 22.3:** Sphenoid bone: Anterior aspect

occupied by a thin plate of bone called *sphenoidal concha.*

5. Each sphenoidal concha consists of an anterior part which is vertical and quadrangular and a posterior part which is horizontal and triangular.

i. *Anterior part*

It consists of an upper and lateral depressed area which completes the posterior ethmoidal sinus and articulates below with the orbital process of palatine bone. Its lower and medial part forms part of the roof of the nasal cavity and is perforated above by the round opening through which sphenoidal sinus communicates with sphenoethmoidal recess of nasal cavity.

ii. *Posterior part*

It forms part of the roof of nasal cavity and completes the *sphenopalatine foramen.*

d. Lateral surface

1. Its lower part unites with the greater wing and medial pterygoid plate.

2. Its upper part is marked by *carotid sulcus* which lodges internal caroid artery and cavernous sinus.

3. The lateral margin of the carotid sulcus at its posterior end, projects backwards into tongue shaped *lingula*.

4. Lingula lies just above the posterior opening of *pterygoid canal*.

### B. Sphenoidal sinuses

1. These are two large air spaces present in the body of sphenoid.

2. The two sinuses are separated by a septum and are rarely symmetrical.

3. *Relations*

Superiorly – Optic chiasma.
– Pituitary gland.

Laterally – Internal carotid artery.
– Cavernous sinus.

4. *Size*

Vertical height: 2 cm (little less then 2 cm)

Transverse breadth: 1.8 cm

Anteroposterior depth: 2.1 cm (little more than 2 cm).

**Note:** *For simplification students may consider all the measurements approximately as 2 cm.*

5. Each sinus communicates with the spheno-ethmoidal recess.

6. *Development*

i. Sphenoidal sinus starts developing as nasal mucosal evagination during intrauterine life.

ii. These are in the form of minute cavities at birth.

iii. It develops to its adult size in adolescence.

## II. Wings

### A. Greater wings

There are two greater wings, a right and a left. Each has three surfaces (cerebral, lateral and orbital) and several margins.

#### a. Surfaces

##### i. Cerebral surface

It is concave. It forms part of middle cranial fossa. It is related to temporal lobe of cerebrum. It possesses following foramina.

1. *Foramen rotundum*

It is situated in the anteromedial part. *Maxillary nerve* passes through it.

2. *Foramen ovale*

It is situated posterolateral to foramen rotundum. It transmits:

– *Mandibular nerve.*

– *Accessory meningeal artery.*

– *Lesser petrosal nerve.*

– *Emissary vein.*

**Note:** *Remember, it is the MALE which passes through foramen ovale in which M—Mandibular nerve, A—Accessory meningeal artery, L—Lesser petrosal nerve E—Emissary vein.*

3. *Emissary sphenoidal foramen*

It is an inconstant foramen present medial to foramen ovale. It transmits *emissary vein.*

4. *Foramen spinosum*

It is lateral to foramen ovale. It transmits:

– *Middle meningeal artery.*

– *Nervus spinosus.*

5. *Canaliculus innominatus*

It is occasionally present between foramen ovale and foramen spinosum. If present, it transmits *lesser petrosal nerve.*

##### ii. Lateral surface

1. It is convex from above downwards.

2. *Infratemporal crest* is an anteroposterior ridge which divides the lateral surface into an upper *temporal* and a lower *infratemporal parts.*

3. *Temporal surface* forms part of temporal fossa and gives origin to *temporalis muscle.*

4. *Infratemporal surface* forms roof of infratemporal fossa and gives origin to *upper head of lateral pterygoid muscle.* This surface possesses openings of *foramen ovale* and *foramen spinosum.*

5. *Spine of sphenoid* is a projection at the posterior end of lateral surface. It shows following relations and attachments:

   – Tip gives attachment to *sphenomandibular ligament.*

   – Medially it is related to *chorda tympani nerve* and *auditory tube.*

   – Laterally it is related to *auriculotemporal nerve.*

### iii. Orbital surface

1. It is quadrilateral in shape.

2. It forms posterior part of the lateral wall of orbit.

3. Its upper serrated edge articulates with orbital plate of frontal bone.

4. Its lateral serrated margin articulates with zygomatic bone.

5. Its inferior smooth border forms the posterolateral boundary of *inferior orbital fissure.*

6. Its medial sharp margin constitutes lower boundary of *superior orbital fissure.* A projection from this border provides attachment to *common tendinous ring.*

7. Below the medial end of superior orbital fissure is a depressed area pierced by *foramen rotundum.*

### b. Margins

1. The tip of the greater wing is called *parietal margin.* It articulates with sphenoidal angle of parietal bone at pterion.

2. *Posterior margin* of the greater wing extends from body of sphenoid to its spine. Its medial half forms the anterior boundary of foramen lacerum and receives the opening of pterygoid canal. Its lateral half articulates with the petrous temporal.

3. *Lateral margin* extends forwards from spine to the tip of greater wing. This is *also called squasmosal margin* because it articulates with the squamous part of temporal bone.

4. Medial to the tip there is a *triangular rough area* for the frontal bone.

5. Anterior angle of the triangular area continues with a serrated margin (lateral margin of orbital surface) which articulates with zygomatic bone.

### B. Lesser wings

It is a triangular bone extending laterally from the anterosuperior part of the body. It consists of a tip, two roots (anterior and posterior), two surfaces (superior and inferior) and two borders (anterior and posterior).

### a. Tip

1. It is the lateral end of lesser wing.

2. It is situated near the lateral end of superior orbital fissure.

### b. Roots

1. Lesser wing is connected to body by anterior and posterior roots.

2. The two roots enclose the *optic canal* which transmits *optic nerve* and *ophthalmic artery.*

### c. Surfaces

#### i. Superior surface

It forms posterior part of the floor of anterior cranial fossa.

#### ii. Inferior surface

It forms superior boundary of superior orbital fissure and posterior part of the orbital roof.

### d. Borders

#### i. Anterior border

It articulates with the posterior border of the orbital plate of the frontal bone.

#### ii. Posterior border

1. It is free.
2. Its medial end forms the *anterior clinoid process* to which is attached the free margin of tentorium cerebelli.

## C. Superior orbital fissure

1. It is a triangular slit like communication between the orbit and middle cranial fossa.
2. *Boundaries*

   Medial: *Body of sphenoid*

   Apex: *Frontal bone*

   Superior: *Lesser wing of sphenoid.*

   Inferior: *Greater wing of sphenoid.*
3. It transmits the following structures:

   #### a. Structures which enter the orbit

   i. *Upper and lower divisions of oculo-motor nerve.*

   ii. *Trochlear nerve.*

   iii. *Three branches (lacrimal, frontal and nasociliary) of ophthalmic division of trigeminal nerve.*

   iv. *Abducent nerve.*

   v. *Orbital branch of middle meningeal artery.*

   vi. *Sympathetic filaments.*

   #### b. Structures which appear from the orbit

   i. *Superior and inferior ophthalmic veins.*

   ii. *Recurrent meningeal branch of lacrimal artery.*

## III. Pterygoid processes

1. Pterygoid process on each side descends vertically downwards from the junction of body and greater wing of sphenoid.
2. Each consists of *a lateral and a medial pterygoid plate.*
3. The plates unite anteriorly in the upper part to enclose a fossa called *pterygoid fossa.*

4. The plates are not united in the lower portion to form *pterygoid fissure* which is filled by the pyramidal process of palatine bone.
5. Anterior surface of the pterygoid process forms posterior boundary of *pterygopalatine fossa.* Anterior opening of pterygoid canal is located in this region.

Some details of the two pterygoid plates are as follows:

## A. Lateral pterygoid plate

It has two surfaces (lateral and medial) and two borders (anterior and posterior).

### a. Surfaces

#### i. Lateral surface

It forms medial wall of infratemporal fossa and gives origin to *lower head of lateral pterygoid muscle.*

#### ii. Medial surface

It forms lateral wall of pterygoid fossa which gives origin to *deep head of medial pterygoid muscle.*

### b. Borders

#### i. Anterior border

It forms posterior boundary of *pterygomaxillary fissure.*

#### ii. Posterior border

It is free.

## B. Medial pterygoid plate

It has two surfaces (lateral and medial) and two borders (anterior and posterior).

### a. Surfaces

#### i. Lateral surface

It forms medial wall of pterygoid fossa and is related to *tensor palati muscle.*

#### ii. Medial surface

1. It forms the lateral wall of corresponding posterior nasal aperture.
2. *Vaginal process* is a thin lamina projecting medially from its upper

part under the body of sphenoid. A groove on its anterior part of under-surface completes the *palatovaginal canal* with sphenoidal process of palatine bone. This canal transmits pharyngeal branch of maxillary artery and pharyngeal branch of pterygopalatine ganglion.

3. Vaginal process articulates medially with ala of vomer and forms *vomero-vaginal canal* between the two. This canal transmits branches of pharyngeal nerve and vessels.

### b. Borders

#### i. Anterior border

It articulates with the posterior border of perpendicular plate of palatine bone.

#### ii. Posterior border

1. At its upper end it splits to enclose *scaphoid fossa* which gives origin to *tensor palati muscle*.
2. Its upper end shows a small projection called *pterygoid tubercle* which lies immediately below the posterior end of pterygoid canal.
3. *Pharyngobasilar fascia* is attached to its whole extent while *superior constrictor* arises from its lower part only.
4. A hook like process at its lower end is called *pterygoid hamulus*. Tondon of tensor palati winds round this process. *Superior constrictor and pterygomandibular raphe* are also attached to it.
5. An angular process projecting from the middle of this margin is called *processus tubarius*. Posterior border above this process is called *notch of auditory tube*. This process and notch support the medial end of auditory tube.

## OSSIFICATION

1. Sphenoid ossifies partly in membrane and partly in cartilage.

2. Parts ossifying in membrane are as follows:
   i. Greater wings except their roots.
   ii. Pterygoid processes except pterygoid hamuli.
3. Parts ossifying in cartilage are as follows:
   i. Body of sphenoid.
   ii. Lesser wings.
   iii. Sphenoidal conchae.
   iv. Roots of greater wings.
   v. Pterygoid hamuli.
4. From ossification point of view, the sphenoid is divided into presphenoidal and postsphenoidal parts.
   A. Presphenoidal part is comprised of parts lying in front of tuberculum sellae, i.e. anterior part of body, lesser wings and sphenoidal conchae. Two centres appear for each of these components as follows:
   Anterior body—9th week of intrauterine life.
   Lesser wings—9th week of intrauterine life.
   Conchae—5th month of intrauterine life.
   B. Rest of the sphenoid is included in postsphenoidal part. Two centres appear for each of the following components of the postsphenoidal part.
   Sella turcica—4th month of intrauterine life.
   Lingulae—4th month of intrauterine life.
   Greater wings (including lateral pterygoid plates)—8th week of intrauterine life.
   Medial pterygoid plates—9th week of intrauterine life.
   Hamuli—3rd month of intrauterine life.
5. Fusions of different components of sphenoid take place as follows:
   i. Medial and lateral pterygoid plates fuse with each other at about 6th month of intrauterine life.
   ii. Presphenoidal part of the body fuses with the postsphenoidal part of the body at about 8th month of intrauterine life.
   iii. At birth sphenoid is in three parts, a central part consisting of the body and

lesser wings and two lateral parts, each consisting of the greater wing and the pterygoid process.

iv. Greater wing fuses with the body at about 1st year.

v. Concha fuses with the ethmoidal labyrinth at about 4th year.

vi. Concha fuses with the body of sphenoid before puberty.

vii. Body of sphenoid fuses with the basilar part of occipital bone at about 25th year.

## APPLIED ANATOMY

1. In the anterior part of hypophyseal fossa there is occasionally a vascular foramen termed as *craniopharyngeal canal*. The canal sometimes extends inferiorly to the exterior of the skull and is said to mark the original position of Rathke's pouch.

2. Premature ossification of sutures between pre- and post-sphenoidal parts and sphenoid and occipital bones is often observed in *achondroplasia*.

3. Anomalous development of the pre-sphenoidal elements may lead to excessive separation of the two orbits (*hypertelorism*).

4. Observation of the sella turcica and the hypophyseal fossa in radiographs is important clinically because they may reflect pathological changes such as *pituitary tumour* or *aneurysm of internal carotid artery*.

5. Decalcification of the dorsum sellae is one of the signs of a generalized *increase in intracranial pressure*.

6. The lateral wall of optic canal is infractured during *optic nerve decompression* in the optic canal.

7. A *fracture of sphenoid bone* may lacerate the optic nerve resulting into blindness.

8. Basilar fracture of skull through the sphenoid bone may lacerate the internal carotid artery resulting into *carotid-cavernous fistula*. This leads to *pulsating exophthalmos*.

9. Collection of air in the cranial cavity (*aerocele*) may occur if the basilar fracture of the skull involves sphenoidal sinus.

10. Involvement of the pterygoid processes of sphenoid is a constant feature in cases of Le Fort fractures of mid-facial skeleton but the location of fracture depends upon its type. In Le Fort I fracture, the lower 3rd of the pterygoid plates is involved while in *Le Fort III fracture* the roots of pterygoid plates are fractured.

11. Large areas of the body and medial pterygoid plates are clothed in mucosa and, therefore, fractures of these parts of sphenoid may open into nasal cavity or sphenoidal sinus with *potential risk of infection*.

# Palatine Bones

## TERMINOLOGY

'Palatine' bone is so named because of its contribution to the 'hard palate'. The word 'palate' is derived from 'plate' because it forms 'plate-like' partition between nasal and oral cavities.

## LOCATION

Each palatine bone is located between the maxilla and pterygoid process of sphenoid in the posterior part of nasal cavity.

## FEATURES AND ATTACHMENTS

Each palatine bone is 'L' shaped in appearance and consists of two *plates (horizontal and perpendicular)* and three *processes (pyramidal, orbital and sphenoidal)*.

### I. Plates

#### A. Horizontal plate

It projects medially from the lower end of perpendicular plate. It has two surfaces (nasal and palatine) and four borders (anterior, posterior, lateral and medial).

#### a. Surfaces

##### i. Nasal surface
1. It faces superiorly.
2. It is concave from side to side.

3. It forms posterior part of the floor of nasal cavity.

##### ii. Palatine surface
1. It faces inferiorly.
2. With the corresponding surface of the opposite side, it forms posterior 1/4th of the hard palate.
3. Near its posterior border, this surface presents a curved ridge called *palatine crest*. This crest and the area behind it gives attachment to *palatine aponeurosis*.

#### b. Borders

##### i. Anterior border
It articulates with the posterior border of palatine process of maxilla to form *palatomaxillary suture*.

##### ii. Posterior border
1. It is concave.
2. It is free.
3. This gives attachment to *palatine aponeurosis* (the aponeurosis is also attached to palatine crest and the area behind it).
4. Its medial end projects backwards and with that of opposite side forms *posterior nasal spine*. To this spine is attached the *musculus uvulae*.

*iii. Lateral border*

1. It is attached to the lower border of perpendicular plate.
2. Its lower end is marked by greater palatine groove.

*iv. Medial border*

1. It articulates with that of opposite bone to form *interpalatine suture.*
2. Articulating medial borders of horizontal plates of two palatine bones project upwards to form *nasal crest.*
3. Nasal crest articulates with the posterior part of lower border of vomer and is continuous anteriorly with the nasal crests of maxillae.

### B. Perpendicular plate

It has two surfaces (maxillary and nasal) and four borders (anterior, posterior, superior and inferior).

#### a. Surfaces

##### i. Maxillary surface (Fig. 23.1)

1. It faces laterally.
2. Its major part is rough to articulate with the nasal surface of maxilla.

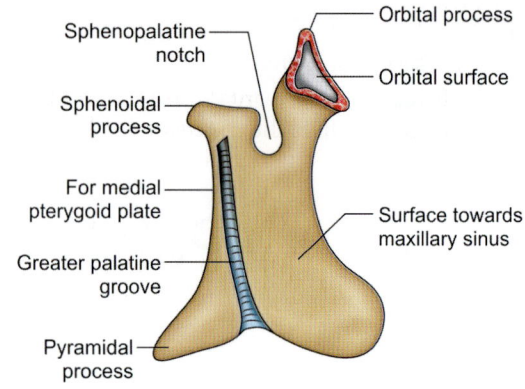

**Fig. 23.1:** Right palatine bone: Lateral aspect

3. Its upper and posterior part is smooth and forms medial wall of *pterygopalatine fossa.*
4. Its anterior part is also smooth and forms posterior part of medial wall of *maxillary sinus.*
5. Its posterior part shows a vertical groove (*greater palatine groove*) which is converted into *greater palatine canal* by maxilla in articulated skull. *Greater palatine vessels and nerve pass through greater palatine canal.*

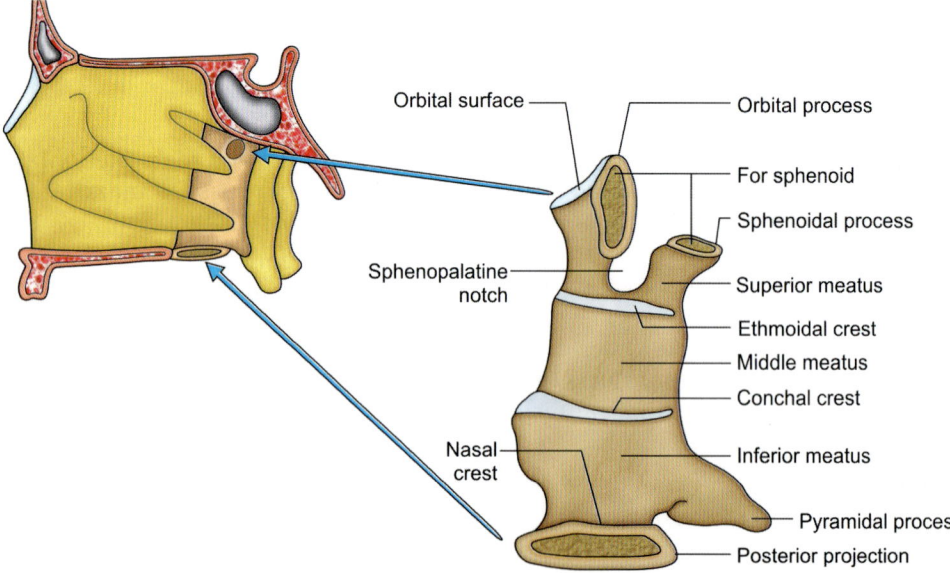

**Fig. 23.2:** Right palatine bone: Medial aspect

### ii. Nasal surface (Fig. 23.2)

1. It faces medially.
2. It has two horizontal crests. The lower crest is called the *conchal crest* because it articulates with the inferior concha. The upper one is named as the *ethmoidal crest* because of its articulation with the middle concha of ethmoid.
3. The area below the conchal crest forms *inferior meatus* of nose.
4. The area between the two crests contributes to *middle meatus* of nose.
5. The area above the ethmoidal crest takes part in the formation of *superior meatus* of nose.

### b. Borders

#### i. Anterior border

1. Its lower part articulates with the maxillary process of inferior concha and assists in the formation of medial wall of maxillary sinus.
2. Its upper part forms the posterior boundary of maxillary hiatus.

#### ii. Posterior border

It articulates with the anterior border of medial pterygoid plate of sphenoid.

#### iii. Superior border

1. It supports the *orbital process* in front and *sphenoidal process* behind.
2. Between the orbital and sphenoidal processes is the *sphenopalatine notch* which is converted into *sphenopalatine foramen* by the inferior surface of the body of sphenoid.
3. Sphenopalatine foramen is the communication between pterygopalatine fossa and the posterior part of superior meatus of nose.
4. Sphenopalatine foramen transmits *sphenopalatine vessels* and *posterior superior nasal nerves*.

#### iv. Inferior border

1. It is continuous with the lateral border of horizontal plate.

2. In front of pyramidal process it is marked by lower end of greater palatine groove.

## II. Processes (Figs 23.1 to 23.3)

### A. Pyramidal process

1. It projects downwards, backwards and laterally from the junction of two plates of palatine bone.
2. It fits into pterygoid fissure of pterygoid process of sphenoid.
3. Its posterior surface completes the lower part of pterygoid fossa.
4. Its lateral surface is rough anteriorly and smooth posteriorly. The rough part articulates with maxillary tuberosity. Smooth part forms the lower part of infratemporal fossa.
5. Its inferior surface presents *lesser palatine foramina* for *lesser palatine nerves and vessels*.

### B. Orbital process

It projects upwards and laterally from the anterior part of upper border of perpendicular plate. A constricted neck connects it with the

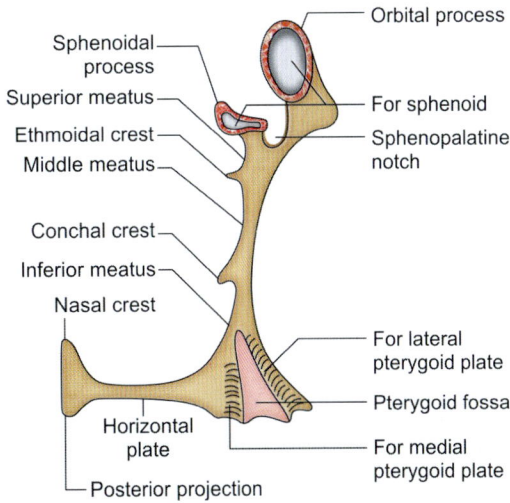

**Fig. 23.3:** Right palatine bone: Posterior aspect

perpendicular plate. It has three articular surfaces (anterior, posterior and medial) and two non-articular surfaces (superior and lateral).

### a. Articular surfaces

#### i. Anterior surface

It articulates with maxilla.

#### ii. Posterior surface

It articulates with sphenoidal body.

#### iii. Medial surface

It articulates with ethmoidal bulla.

### b. Non-articular surfaces

#### i. Superior surface

It forms posterior part of the floor of orbit.

#### ii. Lateral surface

It forms part of the medial wall of pterygopalatine fossa.

The border between lateral and posterior surfaces is prolonged downwards as anterior boundary of *sphenopalatine notch*.

### C. Sphenoidal process

It is directed upwards and medially from the posterior part of upper border of perpendicular plate. It has three surfaces (superior, inferomedial and lateral) and three borders (posterior, anterior and medial).

### a. Surfaces

#### i. Superior surface

1. It articulates with under surface of sphenoidal concha and root of medial pterygoid plate.
2. It is grooved to complete the *palatovaginal canal*.

#### ii. Inferomedial surface

It contributes to the roof and lateral wall of nasal cavity.

#### iii. Lateral surface

1. Its posterior part articulates with medial pterygoid plate.

2. Its anterior part contributes to the medial wall of pterygopalatine fossa.

### b. Borders

#### i. Posterior border

It articulates with the vaginal process of medial pterygoid plate.

#### ii. Anterior border

It forms posterior boundary of *sphenopalatine notch*.

#### iii. Medial border

It articulates with ala of vomer.

## OSSIFICATION

1. Palatine bone ossifies in membrane.
2. Single centre appears in the perpendicular plate during 8th week of intrauterine life.
3. The ossification spreads into the processes and horizontal plate.
4. At birth the height of perpendicular plate is equal to the transverse width of horizontal plate.
5. Length of perpendicular plate becomes double the transverse width of horizontal plate at puberty.

## APPLIED ANATOMY

1. Palatine bone may be involved in *fracture of mid-facial skeleton*.
2. Palatine bone receives adequate blood supply from periosteal arteries and, therefore, all the fragments of fractured bone retain a periosteal blood supply.
3. Palatine bone is clothed in mucosa over large areas of its surfaces. Its fracture may open into the nasal or oral cavities or maxillary sinus with potential risk of infection.
4. *Le Fort fractures* of midfacial skeleton always involve the perpendicular plates of palatine bones. Guerin's fracture (Le Fort I fracture)

involves lower 1/3rd of the perpendicular plates of palatine bones. In cases of Le Fort II and III fractures, upper parts of the perpendicular plates are affected.

5. Horizontal plate of palatine bone may be fractured in uncommon central split of the palate. It is actually paramedian in nature because median sutures (intermaxillary and interpalatine) are relatively strong (Fig. 23.4).

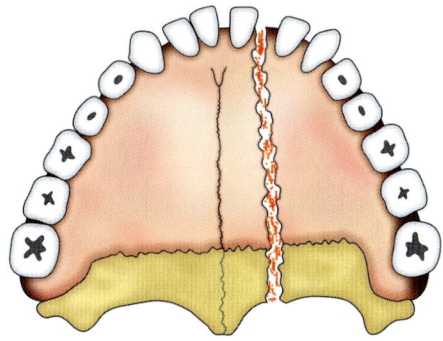

Fig. 23.4: Central split of palate

# Hyoid

'Hyoid' is a Greek word which means 'U' shaped.

## LEVEL

Hyoid lies at the level of 3rd cervical vertebra.

## LOCATION (Fig. 24.1)

1. Hyoid is situated in the anterior midline of neck above the thyroid cartilage.
2. Its body (the bend of 'U') is the first resistant structure felt in the midline of neck, inferior to chin.
3. The tip of the greater cornu (the limb of 'U') of the hyoid can be palpated in the relaxed neck near the anterior border of sterno-cleidomastoid muscle midway between laryngeal prominence and mastoid process.

## FEATURES AND ATTACHMENTS

Hyoid bone consists of a central *body*, a pair of *greater cornua* and a pair of *lesser cornua*.

## I. BODY

It has two surfaces (anterior and posterior), two borders (upper and lower) and two lateral ends.

### A. Surfaces

### a. Anterior surface (Figs 24.2 and 24.3)

1. It is convex.
2. A median ridge divides it into two lateral halves.

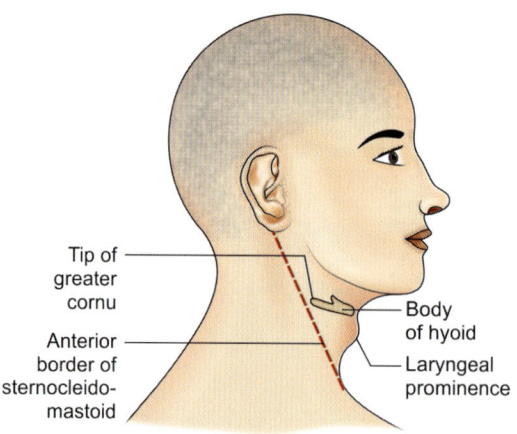

Fig. 24.1: Location of hyoid bone

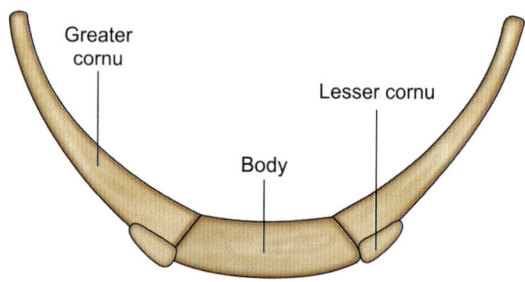

Fig. 24.2: Hyoid bone: Anterior aspect

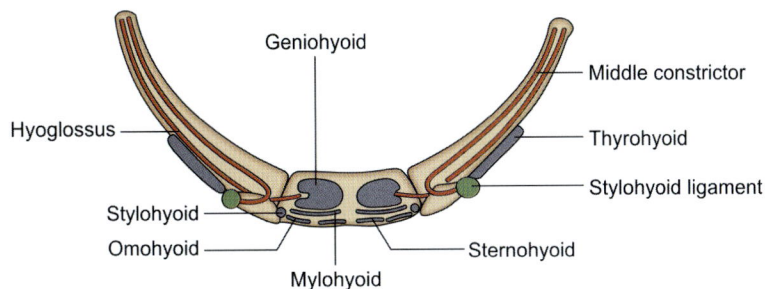

**Fig. 24.3:** Hyoid bone: Anterior aspect

3. *Geniohyoid* and *mylohyoid muscles* are inserted on this surface in its upper and lower parts respectively.
4. *Hyoglossus* partly originates from anterior surface.
5. *Investing layer of cervical fascia* is attached below the insertion of mylohyoid.

### b. Posterior surface

1. It is concave.
2. It is related to following structures (Fig. 24.4).
   i. *Bursa*
   ii. *Thyrohyoid membrane*
   iii. *Epiglottis*

## B. Borders

### a. Upper border

It provides attachment to 3 structures from anterior to posterior
1. *Genioglossus muscle*
2. *Hyoepiglottic ligament*
3. *Thyrohyoid membrane.*

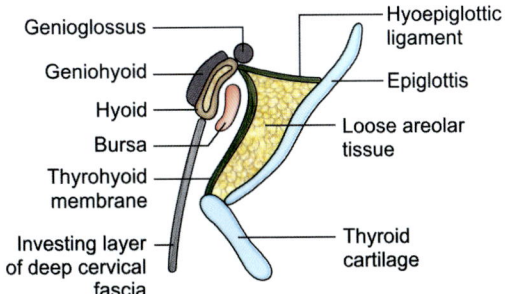

**Fig. 24.4:** Sectional view of hyoid

### b. Lower border

Two muscles are mainly attached to this border on each side of midline from medial to lateral.

1. *Sternohyoid*
2. *Omohyoid*

### C. Ends

1. Each end continues posteriorly as greater cornu.
2. Lesser cornu projects upwards at the junction of the body and greater cornu.

## II. GREATER CORNUA (SINGULAR: GREATER CORNU)

Greater cronu has two surfaces (upper and lower), two borders (medial and lateral) and a tubercle (at the posterior end).

### A. Surfaces

### a. Upper surface

It has following attachments from medial to lateral.

1. *Middle constrictor*—along the whole length.
2. *Hyoglossus*—along the whole length.
3. *Stylohyoid muscle*—at the junction of lesser and greater cornua.
4. *Fibrous loop of digastric muscle*—lateral to attachment of stylohyoid muscle.

### b. Lower surface

Fibroareolar tissue separates this surface from the thyrohyoid membrane.

## B. Borders

### a. Medial border

It receives attachment of *thyrohyoid membrane*.

### b. Lateral border

*Thyrohyoid muscle* is attached to this border anteriorly.

## III. LESSER CORNUA (SINGULAR: LESSER CORNU)

1. It is a small conical projection attached to the bone at the junction of the body and greater cornu by fibrous tissue.
2. It may form a synovial joint with the greater cornu.
3. It has following attachments:
   i. *Stylohyoid ligament at the tip.*
   ii. *Middle constrictor—posterolaterally.*

## OSSIFICATION

1. The hyoid ossifies from ventral portions of the cartilages of 2nd and 3rd arches.
2. Lesser cornua and upper part of the body are developed from the 2nd arches.
3. Greater cornua and lower part of the body are developed from 3rd arches.
4. *Appearance of centres*—6 centres of ossification appear, 2 for body and 1 for each cornu, as follows:
   Greater cornu—just before birth
   Body—just after birth
   Lesser cornu—puberty
5. The cartilage at the tip of each greater cornu persists up to 3rd decade.

## APPLIED ANATOMY

1. Some congenital anomalies associated with developing thyroid are commonly observed adjacent to the hyoid, e.g. *suprahyoid thyroid, infrahyoid thyroid and thyroglossal cyst* (Fig. 24.5).
2. Some times a muscular band connects the body of hyoid with isthmus or pyramidal

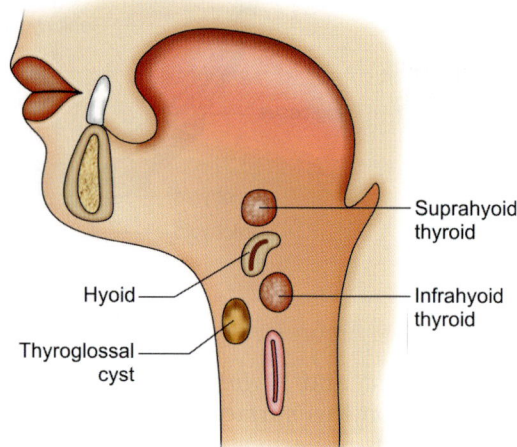

**Fig. 24.5:** Congenital anomalies close to hyoid bone

lobe of thyroid gland. Thus is called *levator glandulae thyroideae* (Fig. 24.6).
3. Lingual artery arises from external carotid artery posteroinferior to the tip of the greater cornu. The latter thus forms an important surgical landmark for locating the lingual artery which is ligated essentially in radical surgery of tongue.
4. The hyoid bone is of great medicolegal importance. In suspected cases of death, fracture of hyoid bone suggests *death by throttling or strangulation.*

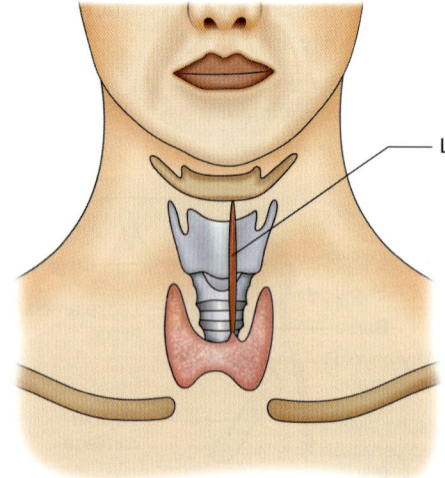

**Fig. 24.6:** Levator glandulae thyroideae (L)

# Vertebrae

## GENERAL CONSIDERATIONS

1. Vertebral column is made up of a number of irregular bones called vertebrae.

2. Vertebral column forms the central axis of the body.

3. There are 33 vertebrae.

4. Vertebrae are named according to regions they belong.

5. Following is the classification of vertebrae:

| | |
|---|---|
| *Cervical vertebrae* | 7 |
| *Thoracic vertebrae* | 12 |
| *Lumbar vertebrae* | 5 |
| *Sacral vertebrae* | 5 (these fuse to form single *sacrum*) |
| *Coccygeal vertebrae* | 4 (these fuse to form single *coccyx*) |

6. Vertebrae are mobile or fixed.

7. Mobile vertebrae are called *true vertebrae* while fixed vertebrae are called *false vertebrae.*

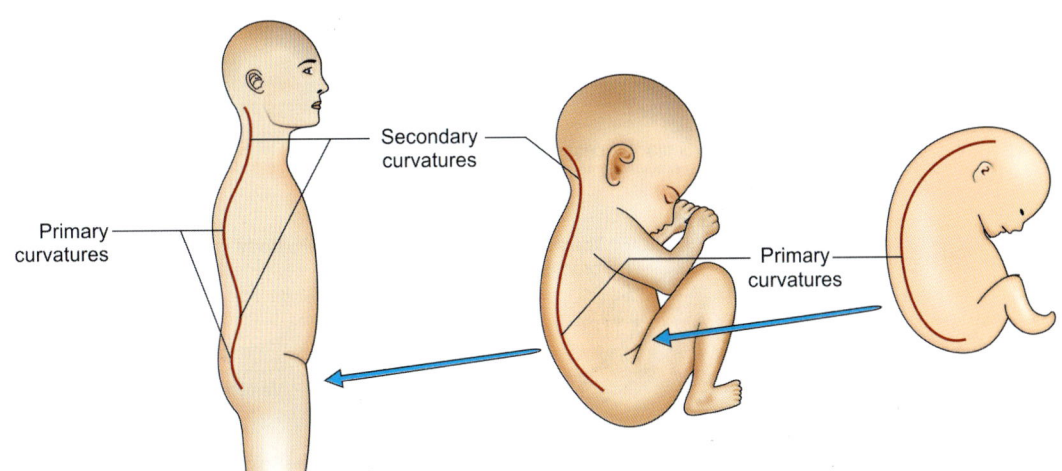

**Fig. 25.1:** Curvatures of vertebral column

8. Movable vertebrae are cervical, thoracic and lumbar.

9. Sacral and coccygeal vertebrae are immobile.

## CURVATURES OF VERTEBRAL COLUMN (Fig. 25.1)

### a. Primary curvatures

1. During intrauterine life the whole vertebral column is concave ventrally and convex dorsally. This is *primary curvature*.

2. In adult primary curvatures are retained only in thoracic and sacral regions.

3. These are mainly due to the shape of vertebrae.

### b. Secondary curvatures

1. Secondary curvatures are convex forwards.

2. These develop after birth.

3. These develop due to posture.

4. These are mainly due to the shape of intervertebral discs.

5. Secondary curvatures are observed in cervical and lumbar regions.

6. Cervical curvature appears around 6–9 months when the child starts holding his head by himself.

7. Lumbar curvature appears at about 12–18 months when the child starts walking.

## MOVEMENTS OF VERTEBRAL COLUMN

Vertebral column shows following movements:

1. *Flexion*: Forward bending.

2. *Extension*: Backward bending.

3. *Lateral flexion*: Side bending.

4. *Rotation*: Twisting of trunk.

5. *Circumduction*: Combination of all the above movements.

## FEATURES OF A TYPICAL VERTEBRA (Fig. 25.2)

A typical vertebra is made up of 2 parts, *body* and *vertebral arch*.

### a. Body

1. It is ventral part of a vertebra.

2. It is cylindrical in shape.

3. It has four surfaces, anterior, posterior, superior and inferior.

4. Anterior surface is convex from side to side and concave from above downwards.

5. Posterior surface is slightly concave from side to side but flat from above downwards. It has number of foramina for exit of *basivertebral veins*. It forms anterior boundary of vertebral foramen.

6. Upper and lower surfaces are rough for the intervertebral discs.

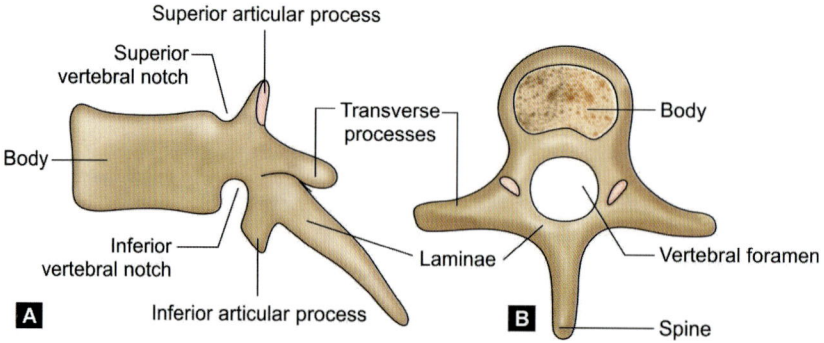

**Fig. 25.2:** A typical vertebra. (A) Left lateral view; (B) Superior view

## b. Vertebral arch

It consists of a pair of pedicles, a pair of laminae and seven processes (one spinous, four articular and two transverse).

### i. Pedicles

1. These are pair of short thick processes which project backwards from the body.
2. Between the adjacent pedicles are *intervertebral foramina*.

### ii. Laminae

1. These are bony plates extending backwards and medially from posterior end of the pedicles.
2. Posteriorly they fuse to form spine in the midline.
3. Body, pedicles and laminae together enclose the foramen of vertebra called *vertebral foramen*.

### iii. Transverse process

It projects laterally on each side from the junction of pedicle and lamina.

### iv. Articular processes

1. These are two on each side and four in total.
2. These are *superior and inferior articular processes* projecting upwards and downwards respectively from the junction of pedicle and lamina.

### v. Spinous process (spine)

It projects backwards in the midline from the meeting point of laminae.

## DISTINGUISHING FEATURES (Fig. 25.3)

1. *Cervical vertebra* is characterized by the presence of a foramen in each transverse process. This foramen is named as *foramen transversarium*.
2. *Thoracic vertebra* is recognized by the presence of *costal facets* on the sides of body.
3. *Lumbar vertebra* is larger in size and lacks both *foramen transversarium* as well as *costal facets*.
4. There is no isolated sacral vertebra. Five *sacral vertebrae* fuse to form single piece of triangular and curved **sacrum**.
5. Similarly there is no isolated coccygeal vertebra. Four *coccygeal vertebrae* fuse to form single piece of **coccyx**. Coccyx is relatively very small in size than sacrum.

## REGIONAL VERTEBRAE

### I. CERVICAL VERTEBRAE

These are classified as *typical* and *atypical*. 3rd to 6th cervical vertebrae are typical. 1st, 2nd and 7th cervical vertebrae are atypical.

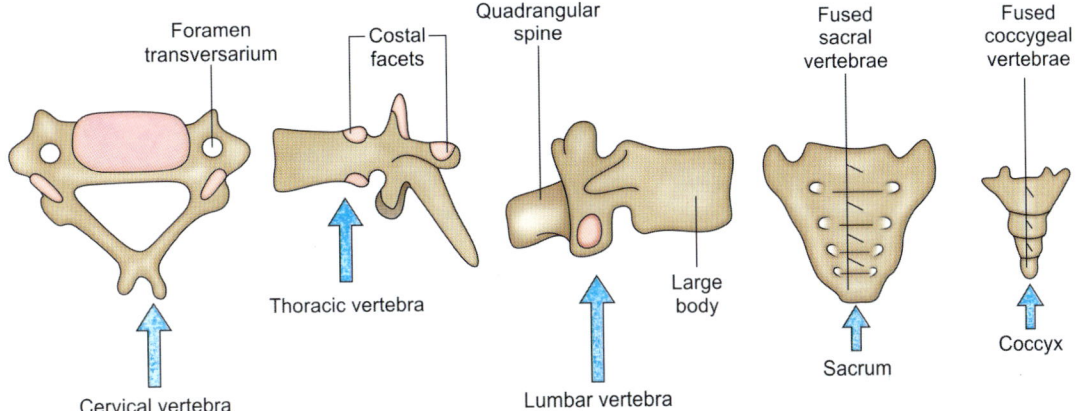

**Fig. 25.3:** Distinguishing features of vertebrae

## A. Typical cervical vertebra (Fig. 25.4)

It has a *body* and a *vertebral arch*. These enclose a *vertebral foramen*.

### a. Body

1. It is smallest among all vertebrae.
2. It is narrower anteroposteriorly.
3. It has 4 surfaces; *superior, inferior, anterior* and *posterior*.
4. Its superior surface is concave from side to side with an upward projecting lip on either side. This surface is mainly related to *intervertebral disc*.
5. The inferior surface is convex from side to side. The anterior border of inferior surface projects downwards to hide the intervertebral disc. Inferior surface, like superior surface is also related to *inter-vertebral disc*.

6. Anterior surface provides attachments to *anterior longitudinal ligament* in the middle and *longus colli muscle* on either side of it.
7. Posterior surface has number of foramina for *basivertebral veins*. Its superior and inferior margins provide attachments to *posterior longitudinal ligament*.

### b. Vertebral foramen

1. It is triangular in shape.
2. It is bigger than the body.

### c. Vertebral arch

It is comprised of *pedicles, laminae,* the *superior* and *inferior articular processes,* the *transverse processes* and *spine*.

### i. Pedicles (Fig. 25.5)

1. These are directed backwards and laterally. It is this direction which is

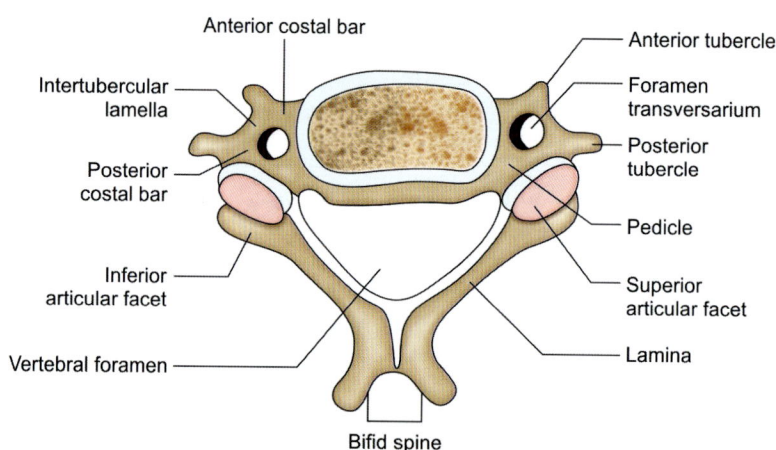

**Fig. 25.4:** Typical cervical vertebra: Superior aspect

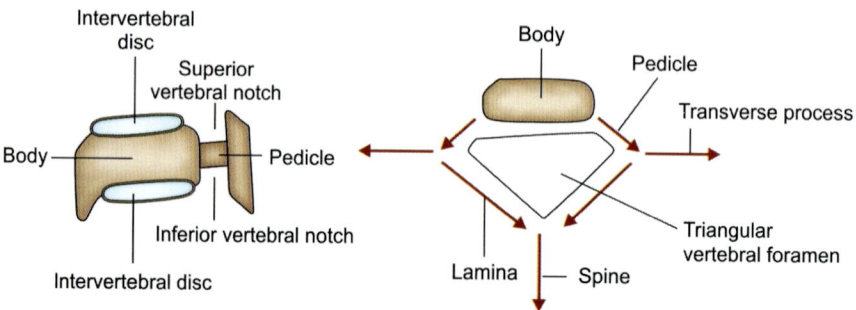

**Fig. 25.5:** The pedicle of cervical vertebra

responsible for triangular shape of vertebral foramen.

2. Above and below the pedicles are *superior* and *inferior vertebral notches* respectively. These notches are equal in size.

### ii. Laminae (Fig. 25.6)

1. These are long and narrow.

2. The superior border is thinner than the inferior border.

3. *Ligamentum flavum* is attached to its superior border and lower part of its anterior surface.

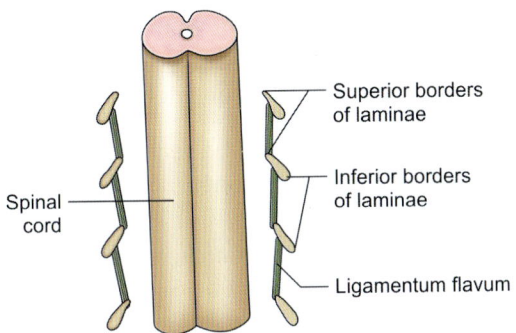

**Fig. 25.6:** The laminae of cervical vertebrae: Cross sectional view

### iii. Articular processes

1. *Superior* and *inferior articular processes* are located on each side, above and below the junction of pedicle and lamina.

2. *Superior articular process* faces upwards and backwards.

3. *Inferior articular process* is directed downwards and forwards.

4. Superior articular process of a vertebra articulates with inferior articular process of the vertebra above.

5. Articular processes lie in one line forming an *articular pillar*.

### iv. Transverse process

1. It has got a foramen called *foramen transversarium*, which forms a characteristic feature of *cervical vertebra*.

2. *Vertebral artery, vertebral vein* and *sympathetic nerves* pass through foramen transversarium (vertebral artery passes through upper 6 foramina only).

3. The foramen transversarium is bounded anteriorly and posteriorly by *anterior and posterior roots* respectively.

4. The lateral ends of the anterior and posterior roots are connected by *costotransverse bar* or *intertubercular lamella* (Fig. 25.7).

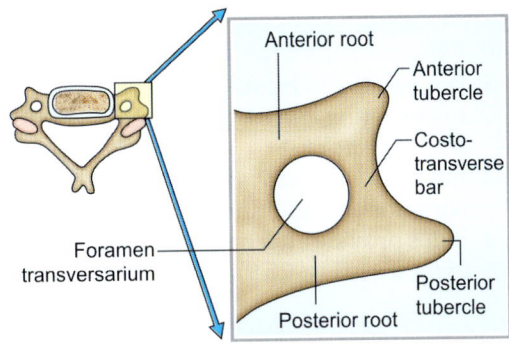

**Fig. 25.7:** Foramen transversarium

5. Junctions of anterior and posterior roots with costotransverse bar are marked by *anterior and posterior tubercles* respectively.

6. The enlarged anterior tubercle of the sixth cervical vertebra is called *carotid tubercle*. This is related to *common carotid artery*.

7. Anterior tubercles give origins to *scalenus anterior, longus capitis* and *longus colli muscles*.

8. Posterior tubercles provide attachments to *levator scapulae, scalenus medius, scalenus posterior* and some *deep muscles of the back*

9. The anterior root, anterior tubercle, costotransverse bar, posterior tubercle and adjoining (lateral part of) posterior root represent the *costal element* while the medial part of posterior root represents the *transverse element* of the developing vertebra (Fig. 25.8).

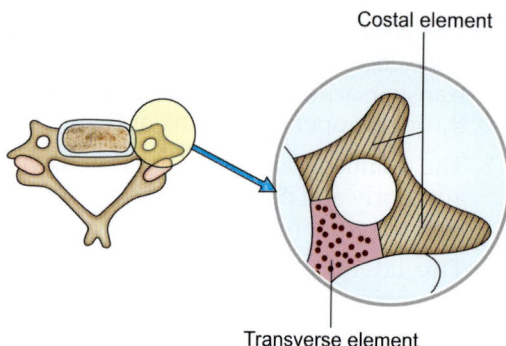

**Fig. 25.8:** Costal and transverse elements of transverse process

### v. Spine

1. It is small and bifid.
2. *Ligamentum nuchae* is attached to the *spinous notch*.
3. *Interspinous ligaments* are attached to its superior and inferior borders.
4. Sides provide attachments to *deep muscles of the back* (Fig. 25.9).

## B. Atypical cervical vertebrae

### First cervical vertebra

### Terminology

It is also named as *atlas* because it supports the skull. According to Greek mythology, Atlas is the God who supported the earth on his shoulders.

### Distinguishing features

1. It is ring shaped with narrow anterior and posterior arches.
2. It has no body.
3. It has no spine.
4. It has a large *lateral mass* on either side.
5. The two *transverse processes* are widest apart relative to other cervical vertebrae.

### Normal anatomical position

1. Two arches lie in same horizontal plane.
2. *Anterior arch* is smaller than the *posterior arch*.
3. *Superior articular facets* on lateral masses are elongated.

### Features and attachments
(Figs 25.10 and 25.11)

Atlas has got an *anterior arch*, a *posterior arch* and two *lateral masses*.

### a. Anterior arch

1. It is smaller than the posterior arch.
2. It connects the two lateral masses.

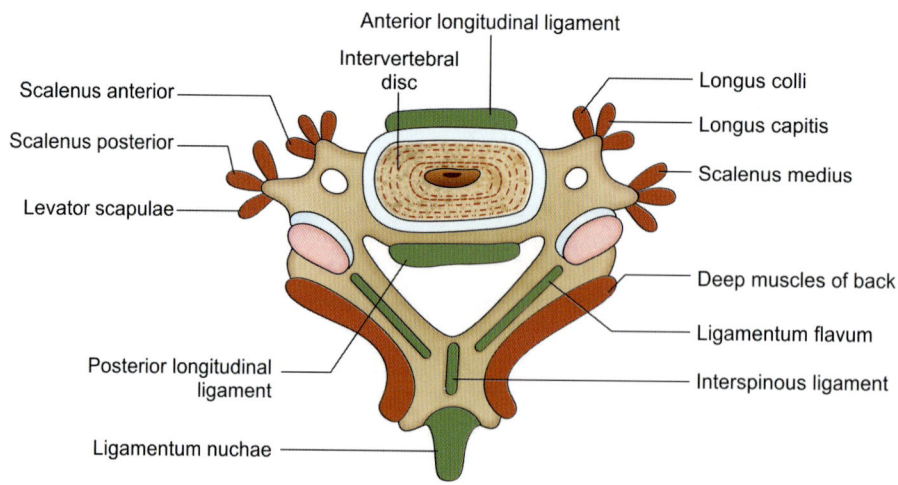

**Fig. 25.9:** Main attachments and relations of typical cervical vertebra

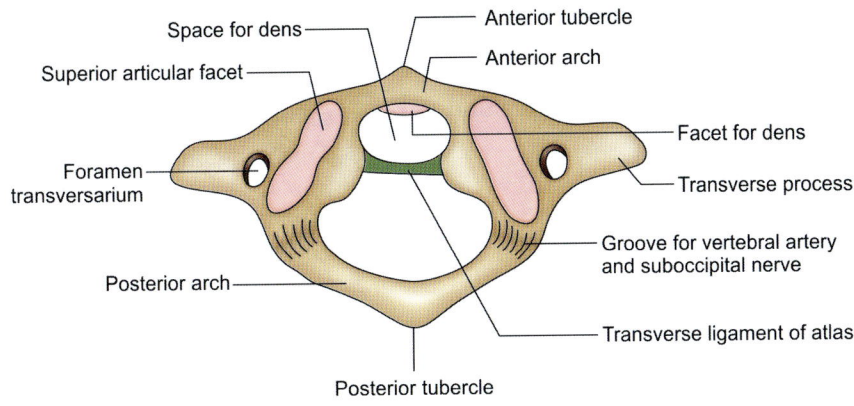

**Fig. 25.10:** Atlas: Superior aspect

3. *Anterior tubercle* is present on its anterior aspect in the midline. Midline part of upper end of *anterior longitudinal ligament* is attached to it.

4. Its anterior surface on each side of anterior tubercle provides attachment to *longus colli muscle.*

5. An *oval facet* is present on its posterior surface in the midline for articulation with dens of 2nd cervical vertebra to form the *atlantoaxial joint.*

6. *Anterior atlanto-occipital membrane* is attached to the upper border of anterior arch.

7. Lateral part of upper end of *anterior longitudinal ligament* is attached to the lower border of anterior arch.

**b. Posterior arch**

1. It is longer than the anterior arch.

2. Midline *posterior tubercle* on its posterior surface represents the spine.

3. *Ligamentum nuchae* is attached to the posterior tubercle.

4. On each side of posterior tubercle is attached the *rectus capitis posterior minor.*

5. *Vertebral artery (3rd part)* and *first cervical nerve* lie in the shallow groove on the

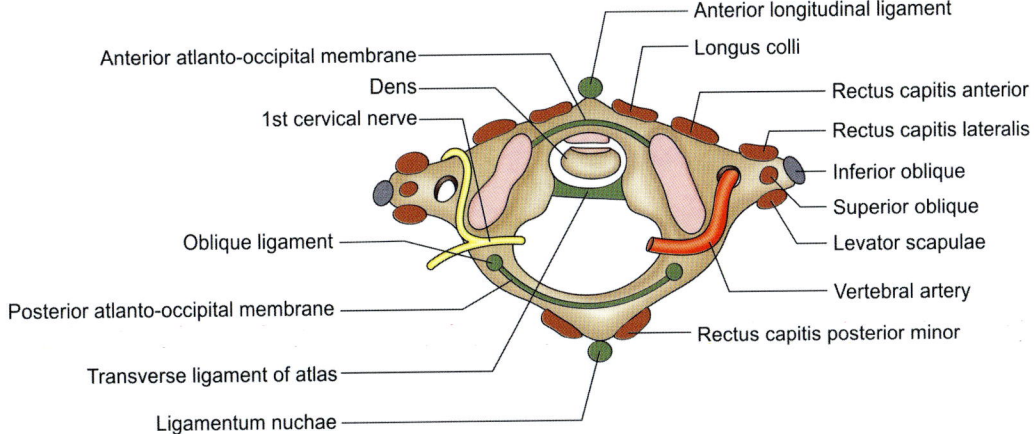

**Fig. 25.11:** Attachments and relations of atlas: Superior view

superior surface of posterior arch just behind the lateral mass.

6. *Posterior atlanto-occipital membrane* is attached to the superior border behind the grooves.

7. *Ligamentum flavum* is attached to its lower border on each side of midline.

c. *Lateral masses*

Each lateral mass has got two articular facets (superior and inferior), two surfaces (anterior and medial) and a transverse process.

1. *Superior articular facet* is concave and elongated. It articulates with occipital condyle to from *atlanto-occipital joint*.

**Note:** *Remember, we say 'No' at atlanto-axial joint, i.e. move the head from side to side while we say 'Yes' at atlanto-occipital joint, i.e. perform nodding movement of the head.*

2. *Inferior articular facet* is flat and circular. It articulates with axis.

3. *Medial surface* has got a *tubercle for transverse ligament of atlas.*

4. *Anterior surface* gives origin to *rectus capitis anterior.*

5. *Transverse process* is long and strong. It has *foramen transversarium* which transmits *vertebral artery, vertebral vein* and *sympathetic nerve. Rectus capitis lateralis, levator scapulae* and *superior oblique muscles* are attached to its superior aspect around the foramen transversarium. *Inferior oblique muscle* is attached to its inferior surface. Anterior aspect of transverse process is related to *ventral ramus of 1st cervical nerve* and *accessory nerve.*

## Second cervical vertebra (Figs 25.12 and 25.13)

### Terminology

It is also called *axis* because atlas carrying the skull rotates on it.

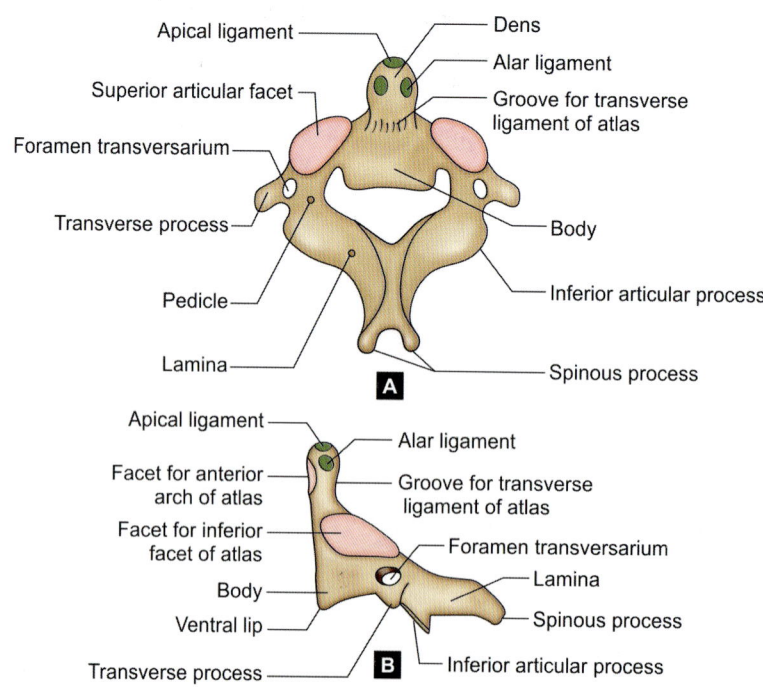

**Fig. 25.12:** Axis: (A) Posterosuperior aspect; (B) Lateral aspect

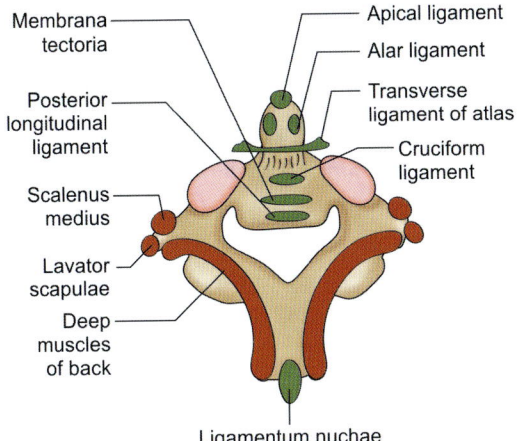

**Fig. 25.13:** Attachments and relations of axis: Posterosuperior view

## Peculiarities

1. It is strongest of the cervical vertebrae.
2. It is easily identified by the presence of an *odontoid process* (*dens*) which is a strong tooth like projection from the superior surface of body.

## Features and attachments

### a. Body and odontoid process

1. Apex of odontoid process gives attachment to *apical ligament*.
2. On each side of the apex, the sloping gives attachment to *alar ligament*.
3. Anterior surface of odontoid process possesses an oval facet for articulation with anterior arch of atlas.
4. Posterior surface of odontoid process is grooved to lodge *transverse ligament of atlas*.
5. Inferior surface of body is related to *intervertebral disc*.
6. The anterior surface of body gives attachments to *anterior longitudinal ligament* in the midline and *longus colli muscle* on each side.
7. The posterior surface of the body provides attachments to following three structures from above downwards:

   i. *Lower vertical limb of cruciform ligament.*
   ii. *Membrana tectoria.*
   iii. *Posterior longitudinal ligament.*

8. *Superior articular facet* (for articulation with the inferior facet of atlas) is situated lateral to odontoid process, partly over the body and partly on the pedicle.

### b. Vertebral arch

1. The pedicle passes backwards from the upper part of body.
2. *Superior articular facet* is large, flat and circular. It is directed upwards and laterally.
3. *Inferior articular facet* is situated posterior to transverse process and is directed downwards and forwards.
4. *Spine* is short, thick and strong. Its tip is bifid and receives attachment of *ligamentum nuchae*.
5. *Ligamentum flavum* is attached to superior border and lower part of anterior surface of *lamina on each side*.
6. Side of spine provides attachment to *rectus capitis posterior major*.
7. External surface of lamina is meant for the attachment of *inferior oblique* in its upper part and *deep muscles of back* in its lower part.
8. *Transverse processes* are very small. They represent the true posterior tubercles only.
9. The tip of transverse process receives attachments of following 3 muscles from anterior to posterior:

   i. *Scalenus medius*
   ii. *Levator scapulae*
   iii. *Deep muscles of back*

## Seventh cervical vertebra

### Terminology

It is also called *vertebra prominens* because it has a very long spine which may be palpated under the skin of lower part of the back of neck.

## Peculiarities (Fig. 25.14)

1. *Spine* is long, horizontal and nonbifid.
2. *Transverse process* is large with prominent posterior tubercle.
3. *Foramen transversarium* is smaller and some times may be absent.

### Important attachments and relations

1. *Spine* provides attachments to *ligamentum nuchae, trapezius, rhomboideus minor* and *deep muscles of back.*
2. *Posterior tubercle* of transverse process receives attachments of *suprapleural membrane* and *scalenus minimus.*
3. *Foramen transversarium* transmits *accessory vertebral vein.*

**Note:** *Vertebral artery occupies the foramina transversaria of the upper 6 cervical vertebrae only*

## II. THORACIC VERTEBRAE (Fig. 25.15)

There are 12 thoracic vertebrae.

## Peculiarities

1. *Articular facets* are present by the side of body and on front of transverse processes.
2. *Body* is heart shaped.
3. *Vertebral foramen* is circular.
4. *Spinous process* is long, pointed and directed downwards.
5. *Pedicle* is attached to the upper part of the body making the *inferior vertebral notch* deeper.

## III. LUMBAR VERTEBRAE

There are 5 lumbar vertebrae.

## Peculiarities (Fig. 25.16)

1. A lumbar vertebra has *massive body.*
2. *Vertebral foramen* is triangular.
3. *Spine* is quadrangular.
4. *Superior articular facet* is concave.
5. *Inferior articular facet* is convex.
6. Posteroinferior part of root of transverse process has a rough elevation called *accessory process.*

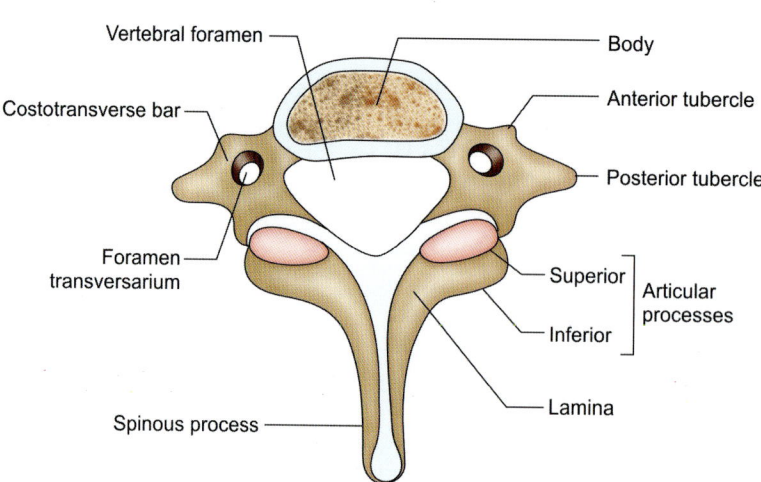

**Fig. 25.14:** Vertebra prominens: Superior aspect

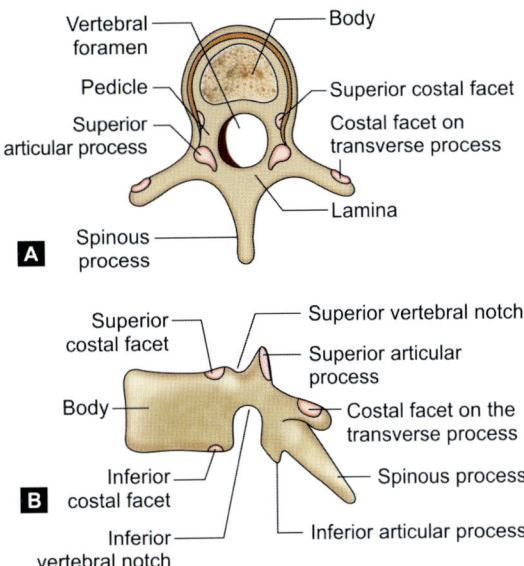

**Fig. 25.15:** Thoracic vertebra. (A) Superior aspect; (B) Left lateral aspect

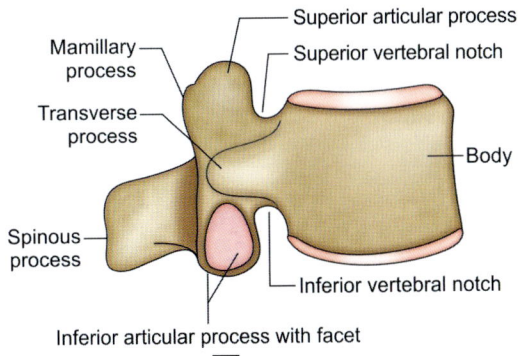

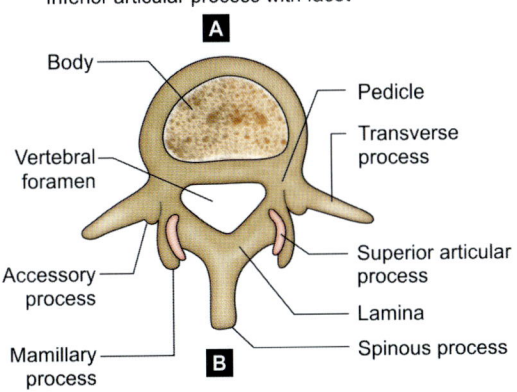

**Fig. 25.16:** Lumbar vertebra. (A) Right lateral aspect; (B) Superior aspect

## IV. SACRUM

### General form (Fig. 25.17)

Sacrum is a wedge shaped triangular bone. The base of wedge is superior and forms the base of sacrum. Edge of the wedge forms the inferior apex. It has 4 surfaces, *pelvic (anterior), dorsal (posterior)* and *2 lateral.* The canal of sacrum is called *sacral canal.*

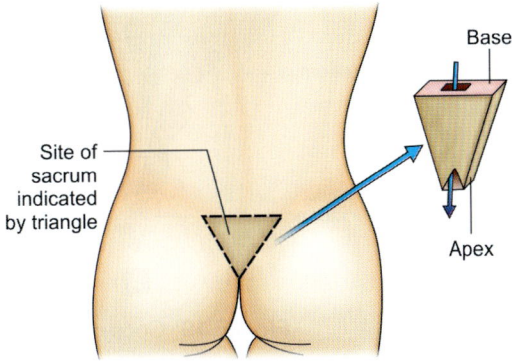

**Fig. 25.17:** Wedge shaped sacrum (arrow is passing through the sacral canal)

## Anatomical position (Fig. 25.18)

1. Sacrum is a midline bone placed between hip bones (on each side), 5th lumbar vertebra (superiorly) and coccyx (inferiorly).

2. Superior surface of the body of 1st sacral vertebra slopes forward at an angle of 30°.

3. Anterior surface of sacrum faces downwards and forwards.

4. The upper end of sacral canal is directed upwards.

## V. COCCYX

### Normal anatomical position

Coccyx is directed downwards and forwards.

### Features (Fig. 25.19)

Coccyx is formed by the fusion of four coccygeal vertebrae. It is triangular in shape with the base upwards and apex downwards. It has two surfaces (pelvic and dorsal) and two lateral borders (right and left).

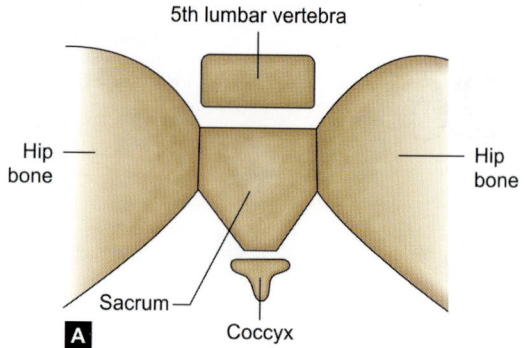

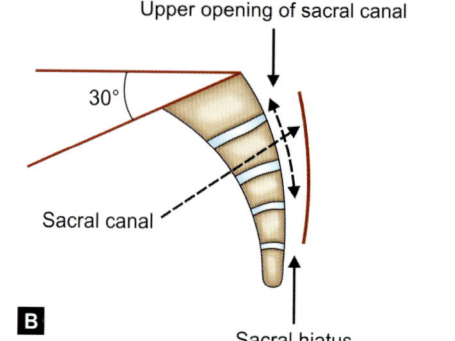

**Fig. 25.18:** Position of sacrum. (A) Posterior view; (B) Side view

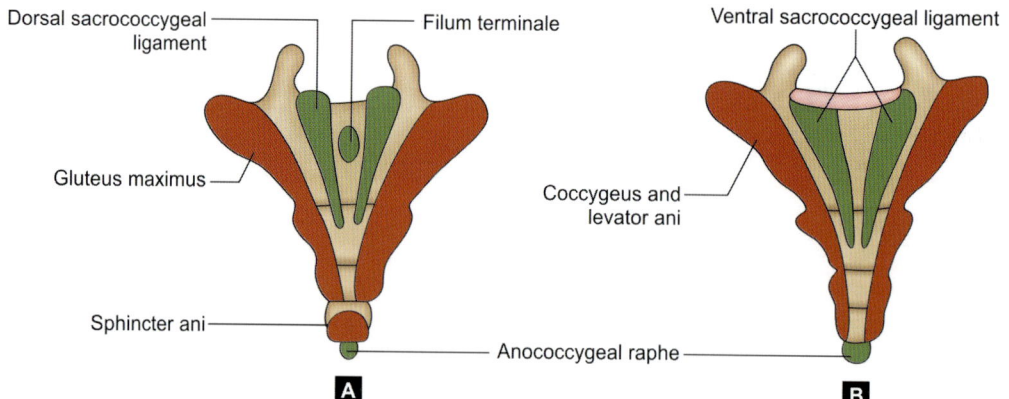

**Fig. 25.19:** Coccyx. (A) Dorsal aspect; (B) Ventral aspect

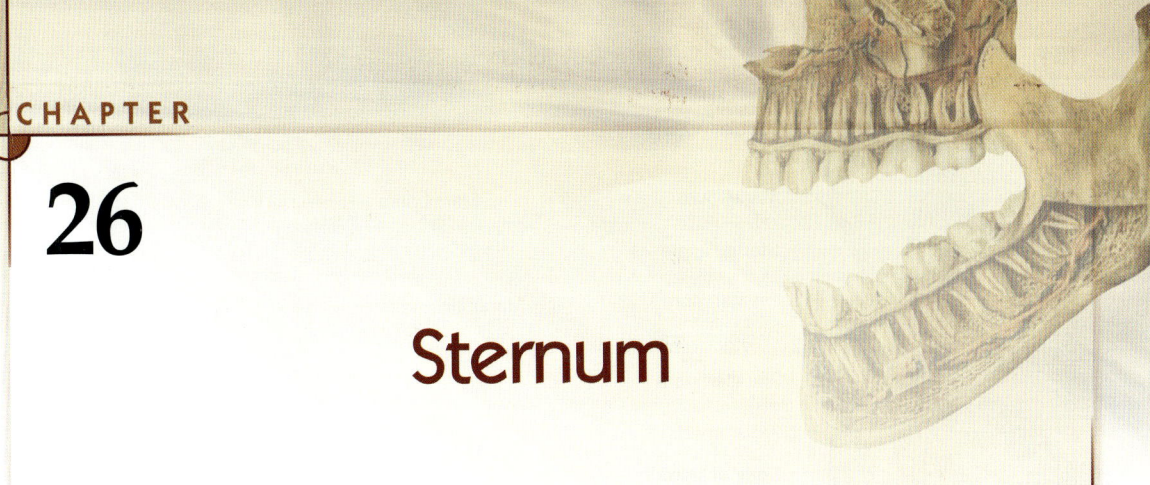

# Sternum

## TERMINOLOGY

'Sternum' is derived from Greek word 'sternon' which means chest. Sternum is also called 'breast bone'. It has three parts; *manubrium*, *body* and *xiphoid process*. Manubrium is a Latin word which means 'handle'. Term 'xiphoid' is borrowed from greek word 'xiphos' which means 'sword'.

## LOCATION (Fig. 26.1)

It is a flat bone whose long axis is vertical. It lies in the median part of anterior thoracic wall. Its surfaces are anterior and posterior. Its anterior surface also faces a little upwards.

## LENGTH

It is about 7 inches (17 cm) long.

## STRUCTURE

It is made up of mainly spongy bone and thus it is rich in red bone marrow.

## FEATURES

Sternum is made up of three pieces from above downwards:

   I. *Manubrium*.
   II. *Body*.
  III. *Xiphoid process*.

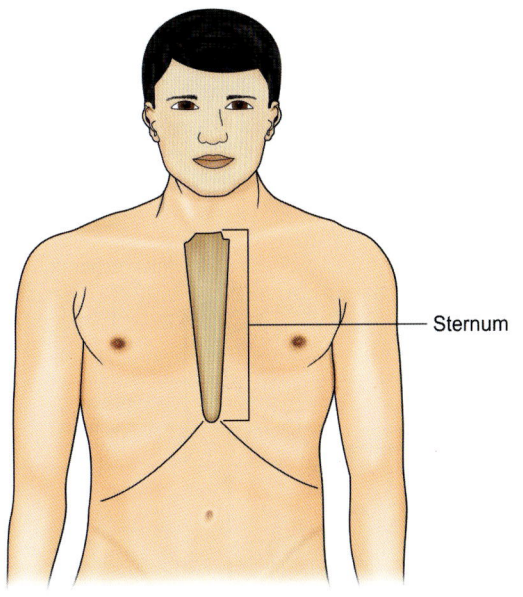

Fig. 26.1: Location of sternum

## I. MANUBRIUM (Fig. 26.2)

It is somewhat triangular in shape and is wider above than below. It has two surfaces (anterior and posterior) and four borders (superior, inferior and two lateral).

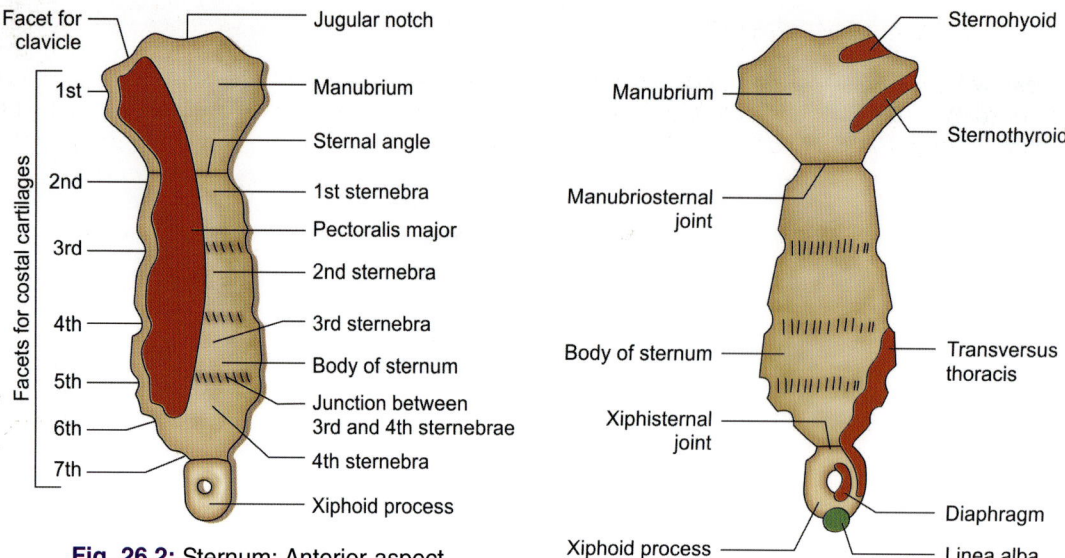

**Fig. 26.2:** Sternum: Anterior aspect

**Fig. 26.4:** Sternum: Posterior aspect

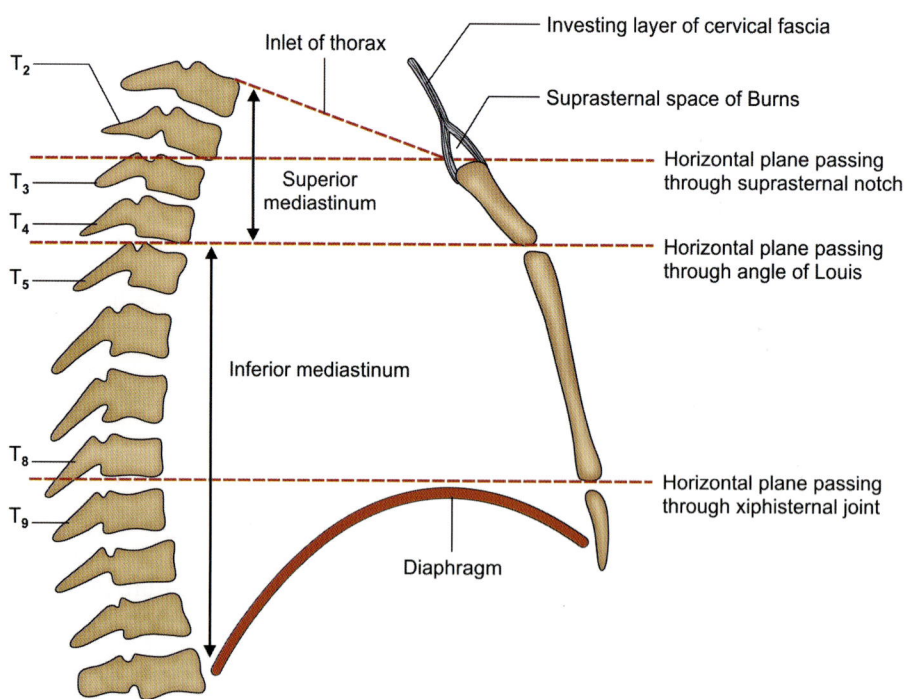

**Fig. 26.3:** Side views of sternum and thoracic vertebrae

## II. THE BODY (Figs 26.2 to 26.4)

It has two surfaces (anterior and posterior), two borders (right lateral and left lateral) and two ends (upper and lower).

## III. XIPHOID PROCESS (Figs 26.2 to 26.4)

It is lowest and smallest part of sternum and is of variable shapes. It has two surfaces (anterior and posterior), two borders (right lateral and left lateral) and two ends (upper and lower).

# Ribs

## GENERAL CONSIDERATIONS (Fig. 27.1)

1. Ribs are bilateral bony arches forming greater part of the thoracic wall.

2. Normally there are 12 pairs of ribs which are numbered from above downwards.

3. The length of the ribs increases from 1st to 7th rib and then decreases from 7th to 12th rib. Therefore, the 7th rib is the longest rib.

4. The ribs are arranged obliquely, i.e. the anterior end is at a lower level than the posterior end. The obliquity is maximum in the 9th rib.

5. The 8th rib is the most laterally projected rib.

6. Width of the rib gradually reduces from above downwards.

7. Intercostal spaces (gaps between adjacent ribs) are deeper in front than behind and deeper in the upper part than the lower part.

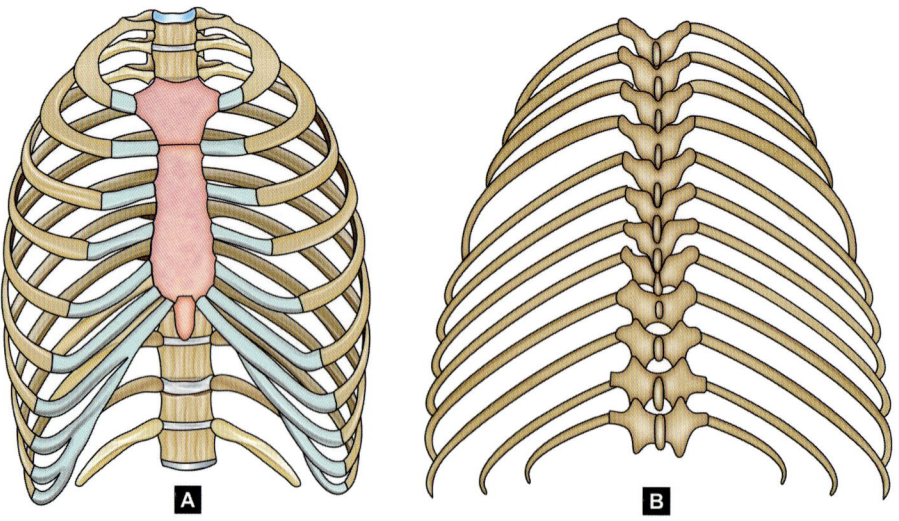

**Fig. 27.1:** The thoracic cage. (A) Anterior view; (B) Posterior view

# FIRST RIB

## Distinguishing features

1. It is shortest.
2. It is broadest.
3. It is most curved.
4. It has no twisting.
5. Angle coincides with tubercle.
6. Head has got only single facet.
7. Costal groove is absent.
8. Neck is rounded and elongated.
9. It is flattened from above downwards and therefore has inner and outer borders and superior and inferior surfaces.

## Side determination

1. Keep the larger end anteriorly and the smaller end posteriorly.
2. Keep the surface of the shaft having two grooves separated by a ridge, superiorly.
3. Keep the concave border towards inner side and convex border towards outer side.

**Note:** *Keep the rib on a flat surface considering its position in your own body. The rib belongs to the side on which both the ends touch the surface simultaneously. If the rib is placed on the wrong side then only the anterior end will be touching the table top.*

## Anatomical position

1. Posterior end is nearer the midline than the anterior end.
2. Posterior end is 3.5 cm higher than the anterior end.
3. Upper surface faces upwards as well as forwards.

## Features and attachments

Just like typical rib, the first rib is comprised of two ends (anterior and posterior) and a shaft.

### a. Anterior end

1. It is larger end.
2. It meets with 1st costal cartilage.

### b. Posterior end

It consists of head, neck and tubercle.

#### i. Head

1. It is small and rounded.
2. It has a single rounded facet for articulation with the body of 1st thoracic vertebra to form *costovertebral joint.*
3. *Capsular ligament* of 1st costovertebral joint is attached to the margins of facet.
4. *Radiate ligament* is attached to the anterior margin of head.

#### ii. Neck

1. It is rounded.
2. It is directed upwards, backwards and laterally.
3. *Inferior costotransverse ligament* is attached to its posterior surface.
4. Following structures form the anterior relations of the neck from medial to lateral (Fig. 27.3):
   – *Sympathetic chain.*
   – *First posterior intercostal vein.*
   – *Superior intercostal artery.*
   – *First thoracic root ($T_1$) of brachial plexus.*

**Note:** *Remember SVAN for the relations of anterior aspect of neck from medial to lateral in which S—Sympathetic chain, V—Vein, A—Artery and N—Nerve.*

#### iii. Tubercle

1. It is large and prominent.
2. It articulates with the transverse process of 1st thoracic vertebra.
3. *Lateral costotransverse ligament* is attached laterally to the tubercle.

### c. Shaft

It consists of two borders (outer and inner) and two surfaces (upper and lower).

#### i. Outer border

1. It is convex.
2. It is thick posteriorly and thin anteriorly.

3. *1st digitation of serratus anterior* arises from its middle.

4. It is related to scalenus posterior muscle in its posterior part while clavipectoral fascia and pectoralis major muscle in its anterior part.

*ii. Inner border*

1. It is concave.

2. *Scalene tubercle* is situated near its middle.

3. *Sibson's fascia* (suprapleural membrane) is attached to it.

*iii. Upper surface* (Figs 27.2 and 27.3)

1. It is rough and irregular.

2. It presents two shallow grooves separated by a ridge.

3. The ridge continues medially with the scalene tubercle along the inner border.

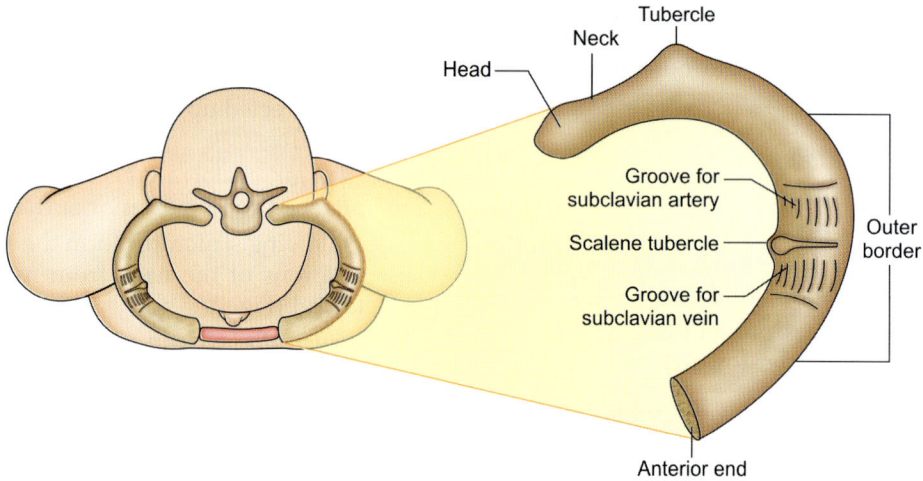

**Fig. 27.2:** First rib of left side: Superior aspect

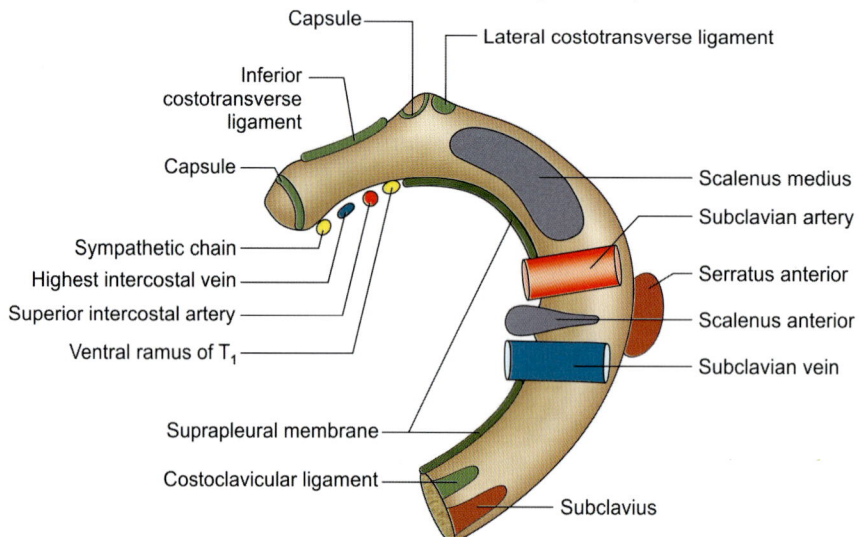

**Fig. 27.3.** First rib of left side: Superior view

4. *Scalenus anterior* is inserted on the ridge and scalene tubercle.

5. *Subclavian vein* lies in the groove anterior to ridge.

6. *Subclavian artery* along with *lower trunk of brachial plexus* occupies the posterior groove.

**Note:** *Remember 'VAN' is the sequence of structures occupying the grooves on the superior surface from anterior to posterior, i.e. Vein, Artery and Nerve.*

7. Area anterior to groove for subclavian vein provides attachments to *subclavius muscle* (anteriorly) and *costoclavicular*

*ligament* (posteriorly). These attachments are located near the anterior end because they also extend over the costal cartilage.

8. *Scalenus medius* is inserted on the rough area posterior to the groove for subclavian artery.

*iv. Lower surface* **(Fig. 27.4)**

1. It is smooth.

2. It is related to *costal pleura.*

3. *Intercostal muscles* are attached to this surface near its outer border.

4. *1st intercostal nerve and vessels* are related to this surface mainly in its posterior part.

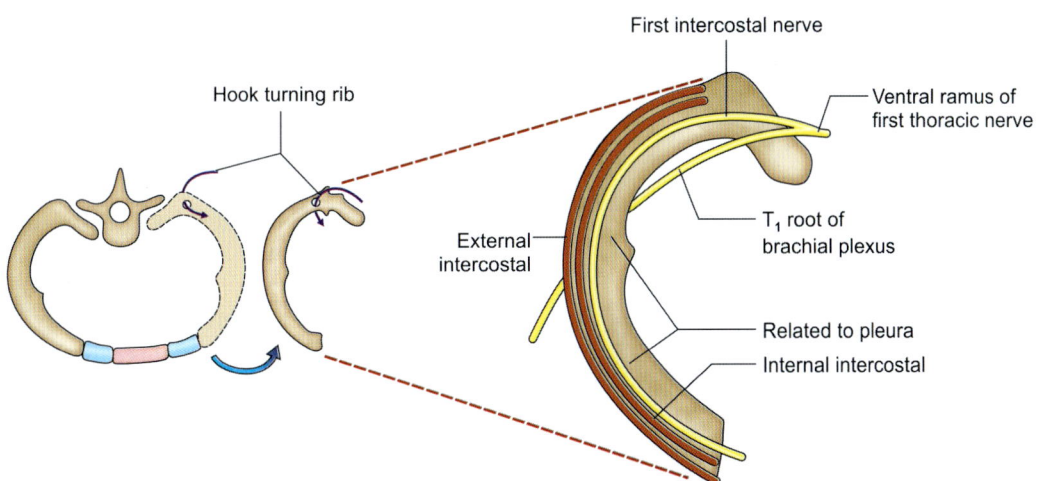

**Fig. 27.4:** First rib of left side: Inferior aspect

# Bony Pelvis

## TERMINOLOGY

Pelvis is a Latin word which means 'a basin'. Following are the similarities between the pelvis and basin (Fig. 28.1).

1. Back or posterior wall is wide
2. Front or anterior wall is narrow
3. Walls are sloping
4. Inlet is above
5. Outlet is below

## PELVIC GIRDLE

It is a bony ring below the fifth lumbar vertebra and between femoral heads. Four bones participate in the formation of pelvic girdle. These are two hip bones, one sacrum and one coccyx.

These four bones articulate with each other to form two synovial (sacroiliac) and two symphyseal (pubic and sacrococcygeal) joints.

## DIVISIONS OF PELVIS

The plane of pelvic inlet divides the bony pelvis into two parts:

I. Part above the pelvic inlet is called pelvis major or greater pelvis or false pelvis.

II. Part below the pelvic inlet is called pelvis minor or lesser pelvis or true pelvis or obstetric pelvis.

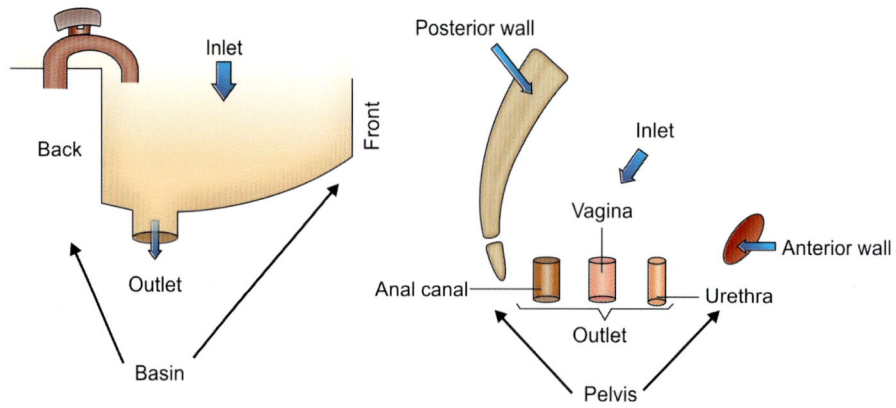

**Fig. 28.1:** Comparing pelvis with basin

## DIVISIONS OF PELVIS

For the sake of description the pelvis is divided into three parts (Fig. 28.2):

    I. Inlet

    II. Outlet

    III. Cavity

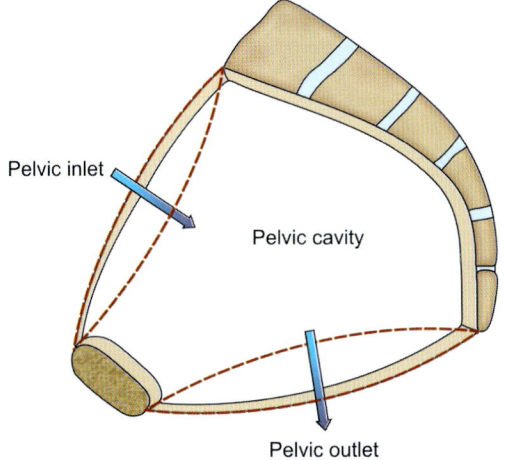

Pelvic inlet

Pelvic cavity

Pelvic outlet

**Fig. 28.2:** Subdivisions of pelvis

# Ossification at a Glance

## DEFINITION

Ossification is defined as deposition of calcium salts in the membranous or cartilaginous background of a bone. The former is called intramembranous, while latter endochondral ossification.

## CENTRE OF OSSIFICATION

The site in the developing bone where calcium salts start depositing, is called centre of ossification. The centre of ossification is first microscopic but soon becomes macroscopic.

## EXAMPLES

Bones ossifying in membrane are most of the mandible, upper part of squamous part of occipital bone, frontal bone, parietal bones, squamous and tympanic parts of temporal bones, upper parts of greater wings and pterygoid processes of sphenoid; palatine, lacrimal and zygomatic bones; maxillae, vomer and nasal bones. Rest of the bones in the body are endochondral in origin.

## PRIMARY AND SECONDARY CENTRES

Though many bones (e.g. lacrimal, nasal, zygomatic bones; inferior nasal conchae and auditory ossicles) ossify from a single centre, majority of them ossify from several foci. One centre in these bones appears first in late embryonic and early foetal life (7th week to 4th month of intrauterine life). This is called primary centre of ossification. Remaining centres, called secondary centres appear later during period from birth to 12 years.

## FUSION OF OSSIFICATION CENTRES

The secondary centres fuse with each other and then with the bone derived from primary centre. The process of fusion begins as early as 3 months of intrauterine life (e.g. fusion between 4 centres of squamous part of occipital bone) or may be observed as late as 40 years of age (e.g. fusion between body and xiphoid process of sternum).

## FUSION BETWEEN ADJACENT BONES

Some adjacent bones may fuse to develop continuity, e.g. basilar parts of both sphenoid and occipital bones fuse at the age of 25 years.

## CLINICAL SIGNIFICANCE

Xiphoid process fuses with body of sternum at the age of 40 years, therefore, enhancing the scope of age determination at a later age.

## CARTILAGINOUS NASAL CAPSULE (Fig. 29.4)

It is the cartilage which forms medial and lateral walls as well as roof of nasal cavity. It plays important role in development of nasal framework. Structures derived from this capsule are sphenoidal conchae, ethmoidal bone, inferior nasal conchae, vomer, nasal bones and septal, lateral nasal and alar cartilages.

Nasal bones and vomer develop in membrane while rest of the above bones are endochondral in origin.

## APPEARANCE AND FUSION OF OSSIFICATION CENTRES

The times of appearance of ossification centre (in case of single focus) or appearance as well as fusion of primary and secondary centres (in case of multiple foci) are represented in Figs 29.1 to 29.4 diagrammatically.

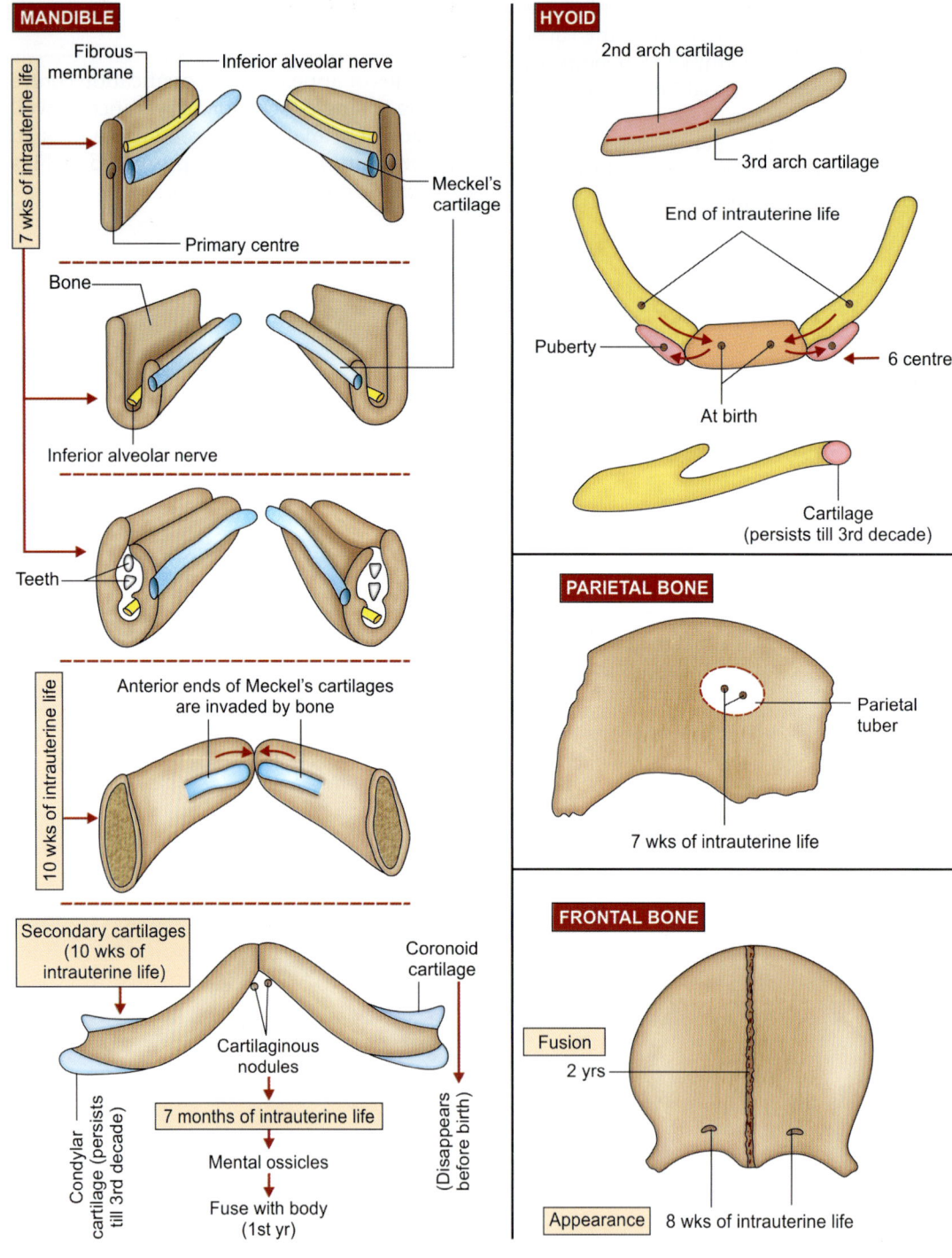

**Fig. 29.1:** Ossification of mandible, hyoid, parietal bone and frontal bone

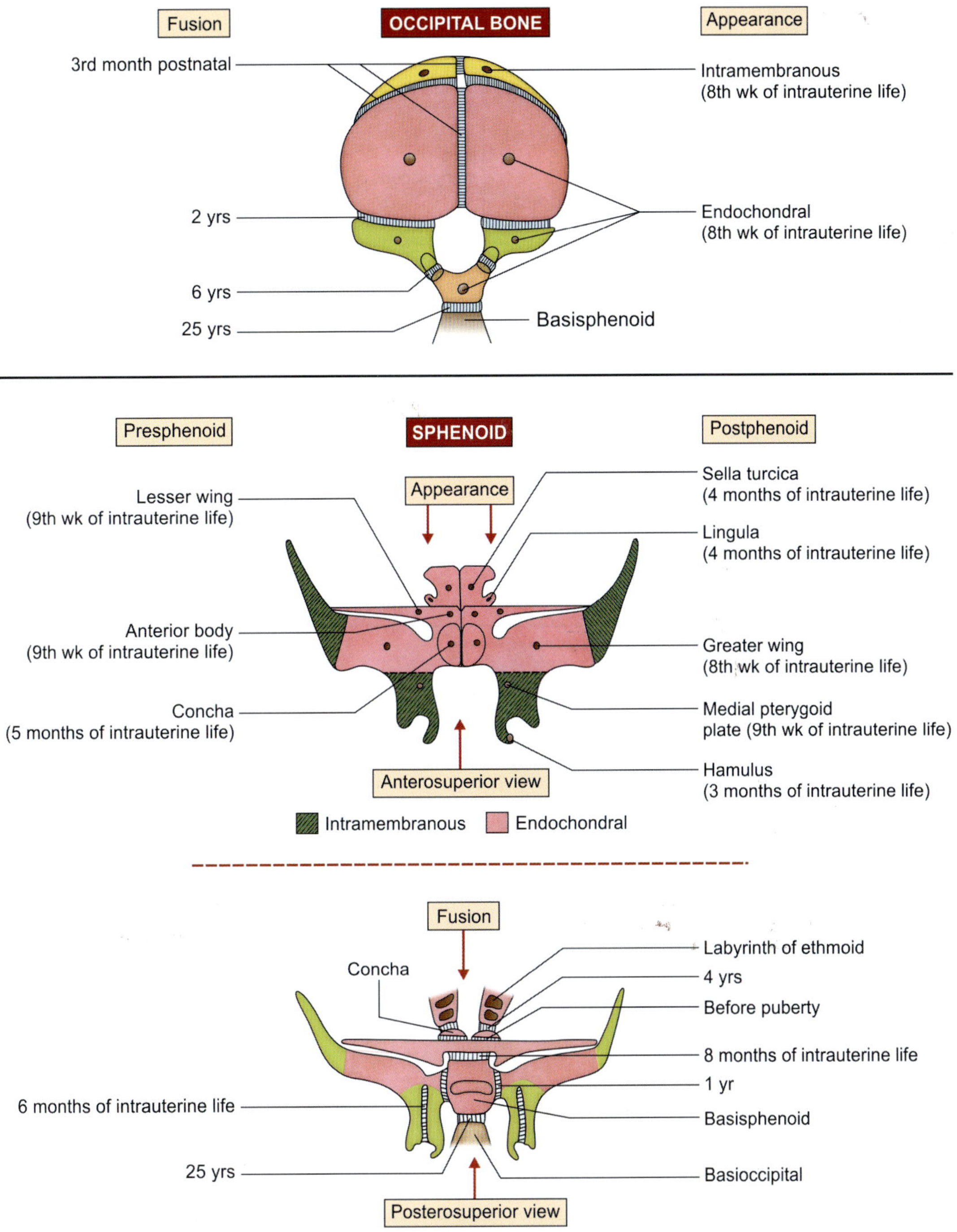

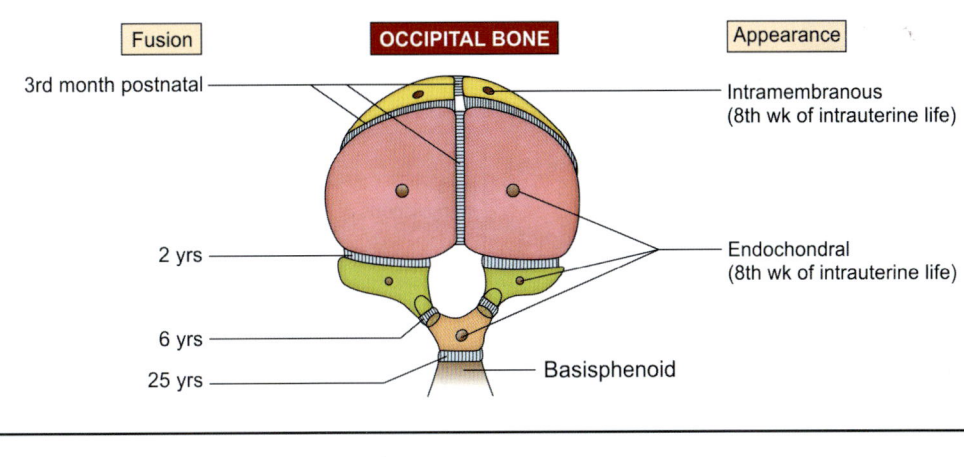

**Fig. 29.2:** Ossification of occipital bone and sphenoid

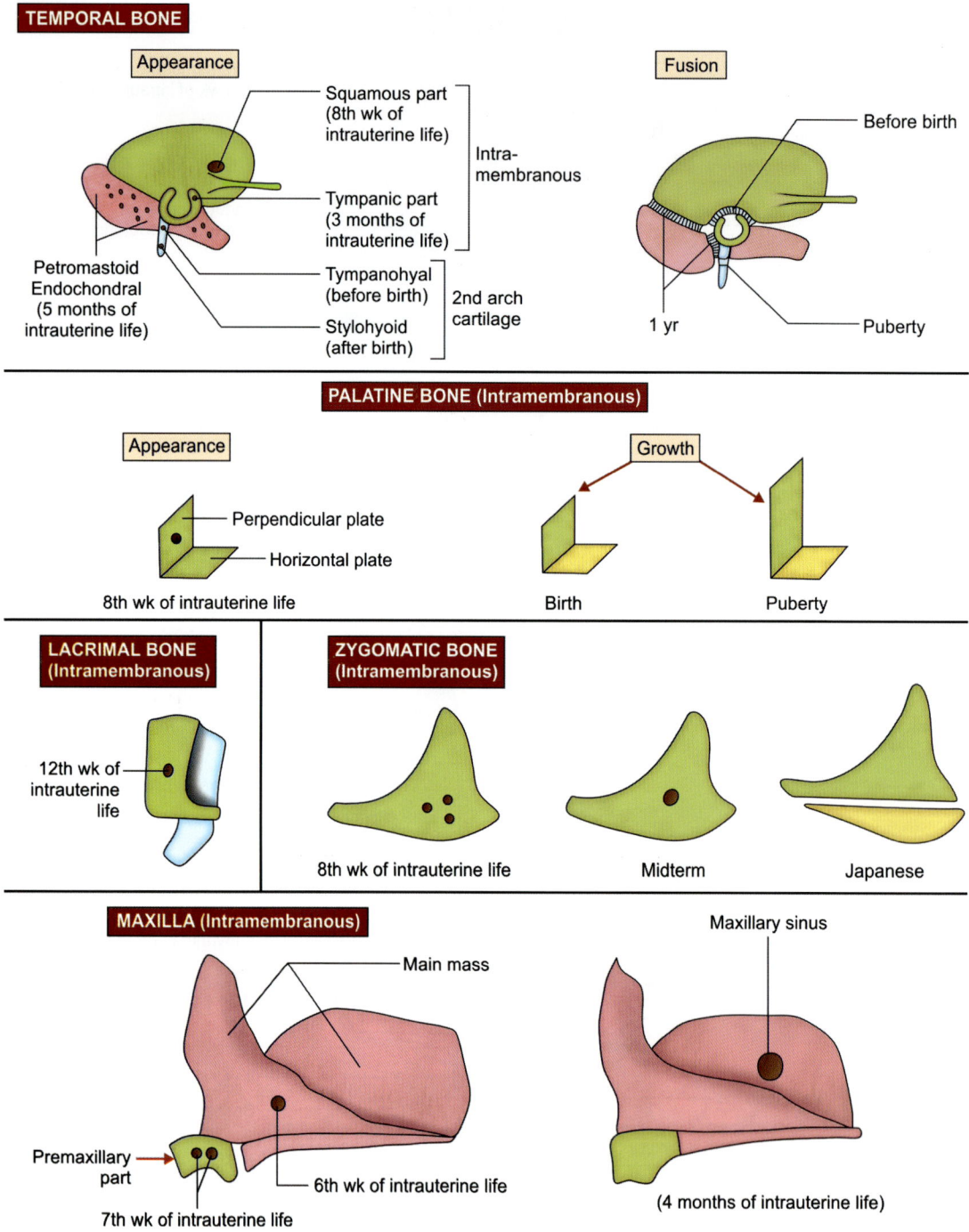

**Fig. 29.3:** Ossification of temporal bone, palatine bone, lacrimal bone, zygomatic bone and maxilla

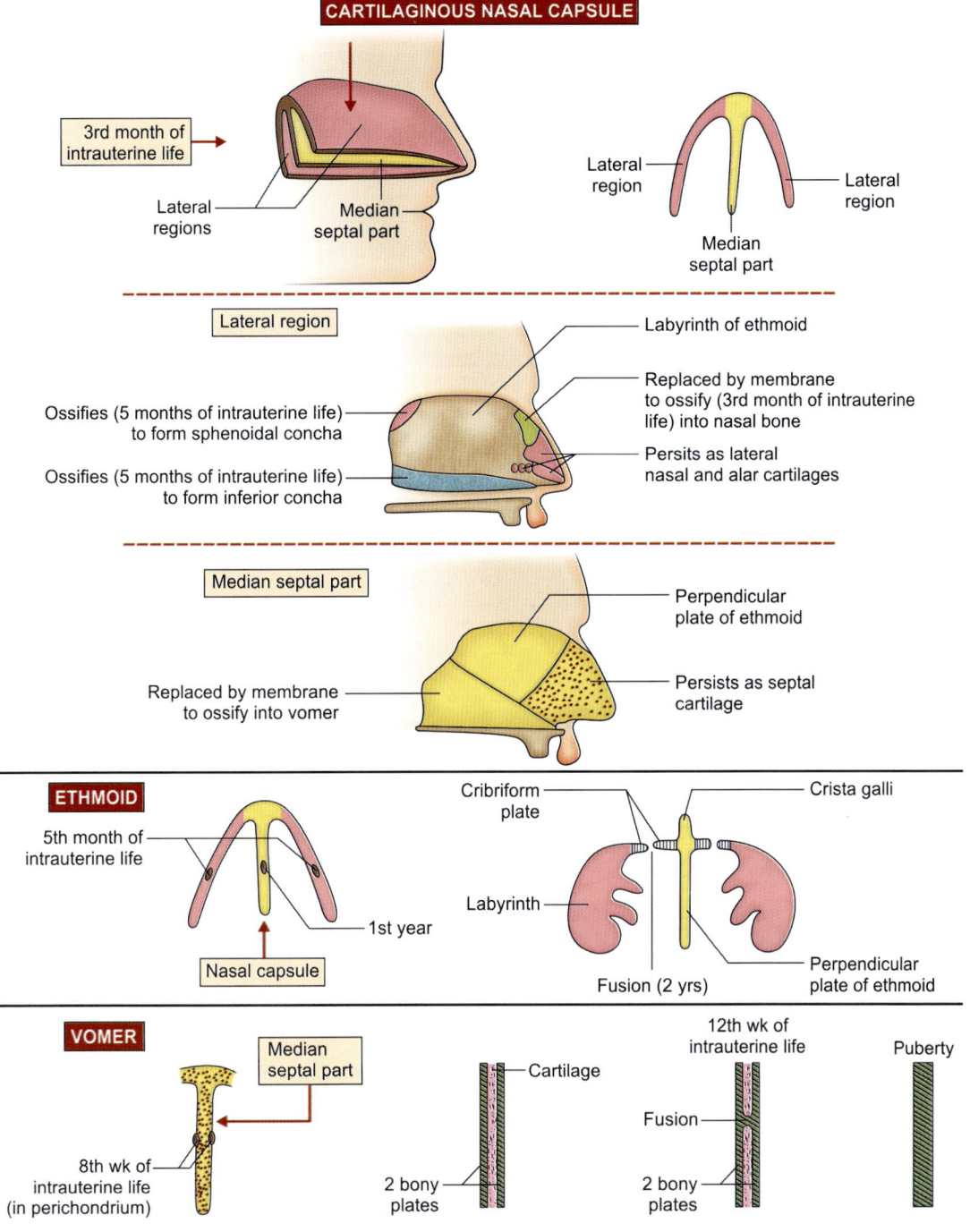

**Fig. 29.4:** Fate of cartilaginous nasal capsule

# Index

**179**